PERSPECTIVES ON AGING

Exploding the Myths
A Lecture Series Funded by the
Colonial Penn Insurance Group

PRISCILLA W. JOHNSTON
Coordinating Editor

BALLINGER PUBLISHING COMPANY
Cambridge, Massachusetts
A Subsidiary of Harper & Row, Publishers, Inc.

International Standard Book Number: 0-88410-734-5

Library of Congress Catalog Card Number: 81-10995

Printed in the United States of America

Library of Congress Cataloging in Publication Data
Main entry under title:

Perspectives on aging.

"The Perspectives on aging lecture series was held at Duke University, the University of Michigan, the University of Southern California, and the University of Washington, under the auspices of Colonial Penn Insurance Group, Philadelphia, Pennsylvania."
  Bibliography: p.
  Includes index.
  1. Aging—Congresses. 2. Gerontology—Congresses.
QP86.P47   362.6   81-10995
ISBN 0-88410-734-5   AACR2

Contents

LIST OF FIGURES

LIST OF TABLES

Foreword

A scant twenty years have passed since John Fitzgerald Kennedy became America's youngest president. His Camelot was a paradise for the young. The mature citizen, whether businessman or bureaucrat, was urged to step aside for the vigorous young man or woman with new ideas and new determination. Older Americans were not forgotten, they were simply shelved.

The election of Ronald Reagan as President—this nation's oldest chief of state—speaks eloquently of society's changing views toward age and the abilities of its older citizens. It signals a new confidence in the elderly, and new obligations.

Indeed, our concept of aging has done a complete about-face. Men and women age fifty and over are now expected to continue active, working lives well into their seventies. Early retirement is becoming as rare as cheap energy. Even retirement at sixty-five is a luxury a growing number of our citizens cannot afford. Second careers are becoming commonplace as older people go back to work.

While the process of aging has not changed, our attitudes toward the opportunities and problems of aging clearly have. We at Colonial Penn are grateful for the role we have played in sparking a part of this renaissance. When our insurance company was formed more than twenty years ago to provide protection for older citizens, we were considered out-of-step with the industry. The intervening years have vindicated our pioneering concepts. Today a large number of insurance companies provide this coverage.

Of our many contributions in emphasizing the positive aspects of aging, sponsorship of *Perspectives on Aging*, the Colonial Penn Group lecture series, is a source of continuing satisfaction. The fourteen lectures included in this book were first presented during 1980 at Duke University and the Universities of Southern California, Michigan, and Washington. Each university has a highly respected gerontological center which has contributed significantly to society's knowledge of the aging process.

The lectures cover a variety of subjects ranging from the prospects for and implications of national health insurance for older Americans to the creativity of elderly black jazz musicians. Some are highly speculative, while others are steeped in scientific analysis. All are informative.

The Duke University series focuses on health insurance, life expectancy, age and the law, and the role of women and aging. The University of Southern California series discusses the use of nutrition to decelerate the aging process, the social impact of longevity, and moral issues raised in the quest to prolong life. The University of Michigan series features creativity among elderly writers, musicians, and artists. The University of Washington series takes an international perspective and explores differing health and social service systems, philosophies of aging, social policies, and cultural influences on aging.

As the number of older Americans grows each year, changes in the social fabric will inevitably occur. We at Colonial Penn believe that research into the aging process and the ancillary problems of a mature population are priority concerns. Scientists, government officials, and business leaders must join in focusing national attention on aging. In some small measure, we hope this book illustrates our continuing concern and commitment to older Americans.

John J. MacWilliams
Chairman and Chief Executive Officer
Colonial Penn Group, Inc.
Philadelphia, Pennsylvania

Acknowledgments

Lines from untitled manuscript poem by W.B. Yeats appearing in "The Continuum of Creativity" are reprinted with permission of MacMillan Publishing Co., Inc., MacMillan London Limited, M.B. Yeats, and Anne Yeats, from *The Variorum Edition of the Poems of W.B. Yeats,* edited by Peter Allt and Russell K. Alspach. © 1957 by MacMillan Publishing Company, Inc. and MacMillan London Limited.

"A Birthday Present," "Kot's House," "Letter to an Indian Friend," "What the Old Man Said," and "On a Winter Night" by May Sarton appearing in "A Literary Perspective" are reprinted with permission of W.W. Norton & Co., Inc. from *Collected Poems 1930–1973.* © 1974 W.W. Norton & Co., Inc.

"The Great Transparencies" and "For Rosalind on Her Seventy-Fifth Birthday" by May Sarton appearing in "A Literary Perspective" are reprinted with permission of W.W. Norton & Co., Inc. from *A Grain of Mustard Seed.* © 1971 by W.W. Norton & Co., Inc.

"An Observation" and "Joy in Provence" by May Sarton appearing in "A Literary Perspective" are reprinted with permis-

DUKE UNIVERSITY AGING IN THE EIGHTIES

INTRODUCTION
George L. Maddox

THE WORST AND BEST OF TIMES

These are the worst of times and the best of times for growing older in the United States. Only recently in his Pulitzer Prize-winning book Robert Butler, now director of the National Institute on Aging, asked "Why survive?" and provided a lot of reasons for answering in the negative. Too many older people are poor, sick, isolated, and impoverished. Our fragmented, uncoordinated system for financing and delivering health and social care for older adults is demonstrably inefficient and ineffective. And still worse, America is an *ageist* society—a society that encourages outmoded, negative sterotypes, shows prejudice toward older people, and is prepared to translate negative attitudes into discriminatory behavior. Moreover, older people not only *have* problems, they are perceived to *be* a fiscal problem. The "graying of America" has produced "the graying of the federal budget."

But these are also the best of times for growing older. The expected survival of the average person into the later years may be a bittersweet triumph in contemporary America, but it is nonetheless a notable triumph. Average life expectancy is above seventy years and rising, and the chances at birth of

3

survival to age sixty-five are better than 75 percent. A great majority of contemporary adults demonstrably live out their lives in some community with competence and, as they report, with satisfaction. Older adults are not, as a rule, isolated from or abandoned by kin and friends. Increasingly the thousands of individuals who, as a matter of social convention, become old on any given day by becoming sixty-five reach their later years better educated, in better health, with more secure income, and with considerable experience in community affairs. For older Americans, the United States is not what it ought to be or could become as a place in which to grow old, but our country is not what it was, either.

Perhaps an affluent country should be able to do better than we have done in adapting more adequately to the aging of our population. Perhaps we should not excuse our shortcomings. But the fact is that all Western industrial countries are navigating in relatively uncharted waters. There are no obvious and certainly no simple answers to some important social questions raised by the rapid aging of a population. Our uncertainty about how to respond to the challenges of aging individuals and an aging society makes us all anxious. The Advisory Council of the National Institute on Aging made the point succinctly in the title of its first report to the Congress—*Our Future Selves*. Construct the future of aging carefully, the report said, because the future you construct will be your own.

A SOCIETY IN TRANSITION

We are a society in transition. That is a hopeful sign in a humane society historically committed to equity and fairness. It is also a hopeful sign in a society whose citizens believe that history is to be made, not suffered.

Ageism and its hateful baggage of negative stereotypes, prejudice, and discrimination are too much with us. Yet ageism is increasingly challenged in conversation, in the media, and in the law. The national commitments to income maintenance, health, welfare, and the maintenance of appropriate independence and social involvement of older adults—inadequate as they may be—cannot be ignored. Nor can we dismiss a growing body of gerontological and geriatric knowledge about aging and about older adults. We do not know all that we need to know. But we know a great deal more than we did three decades ago when scientific study of aging was in its infancy. What we know about the diagnosis and management of disease, about families as a continuing source of social support, and about the organization and financing of health and welfare services is well worth knowing and lays the foundation for realistic optimism about the future of aging in the United States. Our ultimate problem, which we can anticipate with some confidence, will not be inadequate knowledge about aging individuals and aging societies; it will be the development of political consensus about the kind of society we wish to construct as the context for growing older.

THE DUKE CENTER

The Center for the Study of Aging and Human Development at Duke University marked its twenty-fifth anniversary in 1980. It is the oldest comprehensive university center in the United States that has from its inception devoted itself systematically to biomedical, behavioral, and social scientific research and training in the service of older adults. The Duke center has done pioneering longitudinal studies that have contributed significantly to new, realistically optimistic images of adult development and aging. We know that older Americans are more varied than we once thought, more competent, and more resourceful. They have an enormous unused potential that increased social understanding and opportunities can unleash. Duke has contributed substantially to the training of large numbers of research investigators, teachers, and practitioners in gerontology and geriatrics in the past quarter of a century. Its Older Americans Resources and Services Program has produced a model geriatric evaluation and treatment clinic for research, training, and service. And the center has provided its community, state, and nation with a broad range of informational and research support services.

THE SILVER ANNIVERSARY LECTURE SERIES

In universities there is a tradition of "the last lecture." Given the opportunity for a final statement, what significant ideas and issues would a professor choose to discuss? The silver anniversary series of lectures made possible by the Colonial Penn Group provided an opportunity to select four topics of fateful significance for our society. We might debate whether these lectures address the four most urgently important issues for discussion in an aging society. But in our view, they are as important as any alternatives that come quickly to mind.

- Can we imagine an adequate system of health care that the nation could and would finance?
- What are the prospects for—and the implications of—increasing longevity for individuals and for society?
- Does the law, a tool for codifying and facilitating societal intentions and public policy, serve the interests of older Americans?
- What is the new American woman and what is her future in an aging society?

In his chapter, "National Health Insurance and an Aging Society," Theodore R. Marmor conceptualizes the basic components of systems for financing health care and illustrates specific alternative proposals. The proposals considered differ importantly in their assumptions about access to care, about assurance of quality care, and about public and private cost. All the proposals considered, he concludes, tend to emphasize medical rather than social care and tend to make doubtful assumptions about the contributions of medical care to the health and well-being of older persons. To the extent that financing of medical care preempts support of other programs, Marmor argues, the overall welfare of older people is likely to suffer.

In "Prospects for Increasing Human Longevity," Leonard Hayflick discusses with exceptional clarity the current status of biological research on the mechanisms that control human aging and summarizes what we have learned from this research. He distinguishes between research designed to increase the vitality of individuals within the current probable life span (say, ninety years) and research designed to tamper with biological clocks so as to increase the life span. Hayflick seems confident that improved vitality is already evident; he is less sure that a significantly increased life span is likely or that this would, in fact, be a happy outcome for individuals or society.

In "Age and the Law," George J. Alexander argues that a society that is ambivalent about aging and about older people has produced laws that have not served older adults particularly well. The law has, unwittingly or not, victimized older persons. It has, for instance, encouraged paternalistic intervention into the lives of older people that decreases autonomy and increases dependency. The prevailing interpretation of the laws of competency, guardianship, and involuntary commitment to institutions has not served the best interest of impaired older adults very well. In many ways, Alexander concludes, the elderly are victimized by laws that were intended to be benevolent.

In "Old Wives' Tales," Anne Firor Scott provides a social historian's perspective on a notable change in the status of women in our society. It has been nearly four centuries, she notes, since the first women arrived in Jamestown in response to "the heartfelt cry of the men who were already there that they had nobody to do their washing." What have we learned, what can we learn from the experience of the women who have preceded us? Feminism in a variety of forms, she concludes, is one of the few antidotes to aging we have discovered. The biographies of notable American women who made the most of their gender and their age are introduced as cases in point. "So if we can push off," she concludes, "even in new directions, perhaps some historian of the future will be writing that in the last decade of the twentieth century the United States of America developed a new élan, not in spite of but because of its aging population."

1 NATIONAL HEALTH INSURANCE AND AN AGING SOCIETY

Theodore R. Marmor

The debate about compulsory national health insurance (NHI) has extended over fully one-third of America's life as a nation. Since the first decade of the twentieth century, the topic of government health insurance has held a place on the national political agenda with varying degrees of prominence. In the 1960s, government health insurance returned squarely to center stage. The enactment of Medicare and Medicaid represented the culmination of a decade-long struggle about the proper public role in financing medical care for the aged and

Editor's Note: A distinctly new element has been introduced into the discussion of financial support for health care in the year since Professor Marmor reviewed alternative national health care strategies. Stanford economist Alain Enthoven (1980) has proposed a "competition strategy" that features principles of multiple choice, a fixed-dollar subsidy, the use of the same rules for all competitors, and organization of physicians in competing economic units. The recent *Report of the President's Commission for a National Agenda for the Eighties* (1980) endorses a "competition program [providing] all individuals with a flat premium subsidy that would be applicable to a number of insurance and delivery options. It would enable people to select a health insurance plan best suited to their preferences and needs, with respect to the type of health system desired, amenities, coverage, and total cost of care." Although the full complications of the competition strategy for older adults need to be clarified, it is certain that discussion of this option for financing health care will be a major item on the public agenda in the eighties.

9

poor but did not resolve the basic issue of whether universal government health insurance was desirable.

Over this period, the term "national health insurance" has taken on different meanings for different Americans. Some of these different meanings are illustrated in a survey by the Urban Institute of selected national health insurance proposals, a summary of which is presented in Appendix B at the end of this chapter. The political meaning of national health insurance proposals is best understood in terms of scope of benefits and source of financing. The use of these criteria gives us a spectrum of proposals broken into three distinct bands:

1. Narrow benefit coverage, minimal federal financial role
2. Wide benefit coverage, limited federal financial role
3. Wide benefit coverage, large federal financial role

These three categories are illustrated by specific legislative proposals. The cast of characters whose names appear on the proposals changes, and so do the specifics of what is purposed; attention must therefore be paid to the changing sponsorship and content of the proposals discussed.

NARROW COVERAGE, MINIMAL FEDERAL ROLE

Proposals in the first category are frequently directed at "catastrophic" insurance. Catastrophic protection can be provided in a number of ways. For example, former president Carter proposed a national health plan that begins with coverage of hospital and physician expenses after individuals incur $2,500 in medical expenses. The Long-Ribicoff-Waggoner bill, the most prominent example of a catastrophic coverage proposal since about 1974, has prerequisites of a sixty-day hospital stay for hospital benefits and of family medical bills of $2,000 for physician benefits. Other proposals define catastrophic expenses for which federal financing would be available as a percentage of taxable income rather than as a fixed dollar amount of expenditure.

Proposals that emphasize catastrophic protection may provide other coverage as well. Typically this coverage concentrates on discrete populations—the elderly, the poor, or the very young—through reform of Medicare or Medicaid, or the creation of new coverage programs. The Carter plan proposes to reform Medicaid and Medicare and to provide coverage of infants. The Long-Ribicoff-Waggoner bill retains Medicare basically as is and reforms Medicaid. But in general, such proposals leave largely untouched the present organization and prerogatives of the medical care industry.

WIDE COVERAGE, LIMITED FEDERAL ROLE

National health insurance proposals in the second category would provide both wider benefits and broader population coverage. A limited federal financing role would be achieved through distribution of premium costs among employers, employees, and government and through reliance on private insurance companies to underwrite benefits. Plans of this kind can be voluntary (with participation at the discretion of employers and individuals, but generally with government incentives for participation) or mandatory (with all employers and individuals required to obtain coverage).

Many variations in coverage plans and types of government incentives are possible. The employed could have a choice of private insurance plans; the unemployed, either a comparable choice with government payment of premiums or a separate insurance plan. Medicare, or a plan comparable to it, could constitute the separate public insurance program for the elderly.

The mandatory approach to employer-based insurance coverage is illustrated by the Nixon-Ford administration's Comprehensive Health Insurance Plan (CHIP). CHIP would require employers with more than a certain number of workers to provide them with medical insurance; premium liability would be divided between employers and employees in specific proportions. CHIP also specifies the benefits employers would have to provide to their employees. Although benefit packages explicitly require employee cost sharing (deductibles and coinsurance), the benefits would be considerably broader than those in the first category of plans directed at catastrophic expenses. CHIP would combine employment-based coverage with separate public plans for the poor and the elderly to constitute a universal health insurance plan for the entire population by aggregation. The poor would participate in an "assisted" insurance plan, with financing for specified noncovered services. Medicare would continue to provide coverage for the aged.

The Kennedy-Waxman plan, Senator Edward Kennedy's most recent health insurance proposal, is another example of national health insurance by aggregation. Like CHIP, this plan relies on mandated private coverage. Employers would be required to offer their employees a choice of private insurance plans. In contrast to CHIP, individuals not covered through employment would have access to the same insurance plans as employees. Premiums would be calculated as a percentage of income and, for the poor, the government would pay the premium in full. Residual Medicaid programs could also be maintained. Medicare, with some modifications, would remain the public insurance program for the elderly population.

WIDE COVERAGE, MAXIMUM FEDERAL ROLE

The most far-reaching of the insurance proposals within the third category entail a federal monopoly of the medical insurance business. Until recently, such a proposal was annually advanced and supported by Senator Kennedy. Rather than relying on the private insurance market, such a plan would establish a single national health insurance program for all U.S. residents—employed or unemployed, old or young, rich or poor. Benefits would be extremely broad, and patients would not share the costs at time of service use. The plan would be financed jointly by payment of payroll taxes and general revenues and would be administered by the federal government. Administration would go beyond payment of claims to allocation of a predetermined national health budget, by type of medical service, to regions and localities.

With its universal scope, comprehensive benefits, and public financing, a program in this third category of insurance would be similar to national health insurance programs in other Western industrial nations. This similarity, however, should not obscure considerable diversity in financing and administration. In the United Kingdom, for example, the national government not only pays for all services; it also owns the health facilities and employs the providers. In Canada, the national government pays only a portion of total expenses; the rest is paid by the provincial governments which, within certain nationally uniform standards, administer their own plans.

THE ARGUMENTS, OR HOW TO CHOOSE?

The foregoing classification and discussion of national health insurance proposals highlight the primary source of controversy in political debates on national health insurance—the legitimacy and desirability of particular types of government intervention in health care. Government intervention involves such fundamentals as the redistribution of income, status, and influence, and the legitimacy of highly valued political beliefs. Because the stakes are so high, national health insurance generates an ideological intensity matched by few other issues in American politics.

One camp—industrial unions and a variety of liberal religious, service, charitable, and consumer groups—wishes to shift medical care financing from the private to the public sector, in the belief that private financing of medical care has produced intolerable inequities in the distribution of services. They see universal, government-financed health insurance as the crucial missing element in the panoply of social welfare programs enacted in the 1930s. The other camp—ranging from medical and hospital groups to the U.S. Chamber of Commerce and the Young Americans for Freedom—views government financing as synonymous with government control, and government control as synonymous with impersonal and inadequate medical care. They have favored, at most, limited federal involvement in a national health insurance program.

The building-block approach to national health insurance, which has established government intervention by increments of discrete population groups, such as veterans, the aged, and the poor, might be expected to have removed beyond dispute the basic principles of a major government role in medical care. But this has not been the case. As the beachhead grows smaller, its defenders fight more fiercely. The stakes are still seen to be very high, and the last battle may well be fought with the greatest passions.

The intensity of the battle has been compounded by the rapid growth of medical expenditures in recent years. In 1950, the United States spent $12 billion on medical care. In 1977, the national medical care bill was over $160 billion. In 1980, it was over $200 billion. Within the past quarter-century, the proportion of the gross national product committed to medical care has doubled and now amounts to more than 9 percent of GNP (U.S. Office of Management and Budget 1979).

Increases in medical expenses predate enactment of Medicare and Medicaid and are partly attributed to the expansion of insurance coverage itself. Public insurance programs, after all, are intended to reduce financial barriers to care and can therefore be expected to increase somewhat the volume of services provided. Experience with insurance in general, and public insurance in particular, reveals that the price as well as the volume of services rises with insurance coverage. Part of the price increase undoubtedly reflects the rising cost of necessary resources and changes in the quality of the service provided. Some proportion, however, represents a transfer of income to providers, the social value of which has been called into question.

The expenditure increases have significantly affected the debate on national health insurance. Until recently, the issue of cost took a particular and limited form: how to reduce or eliminate the financial barriers between individuals and adequate medical care. Within the space of a few years, cost has become a fundamental political constraint. The cost question is properly framed not by asking, "How can the American citizen secure medical care?" but rather, "How can the American government afford a national health insurance program?" Cost considerations have been used to justify the assertion that the nation cannot afford national health insurance. This argument is espoused by the new breed of conservative Democrats, who join with Republicans in opposition to national health insurance.

The counterargument, made by liberal Democrats and their constituents, is that national health insurance is required to bring the current medical inflation under control—in other words, that the nation cannot afford *not* to have national health insurance. (For extensive discussion of national health insurance, see Feder, Holahan, and Marmor 1980.)

FOCUSING ON THE ELDERLY

Considering programs such as Social Security, Medicare, Medicaid, Supplemental Security Income, and housing subsidies, public investment in the welfare of the elderly is undeniably substantial. No other age group has such a range of costly social programs directed toward it. And for these outlays there are numerous, sometimes conflicting, rationales: (1) the economically disadvantaged status of the elderly; (2) their growing political power; (3) a sociopsychological need to compensate the elderly for the decline in their social contribution; (4) the belief that each generation should provide for the aged and, in turn, be provided for when aged; and (5) the view that the elderly should be rewarded for their past contributions to society (Marmor, Gold, and Kutza 1976).

Although these arguments have continuing support, their weight in the deliberations over national health insurance has diminished as American fiscal constraints worsen. The elderly's privileged position as a group deserving special consideration in government health policies has eroded, or more precisely, been increasingly challenged (Binstock 1979).

Improvements in national health insurance for the elderly may entail fierce competition with other interest groups. If the elderly share virtually the same coverage plan with other groups, advocates for the elderly may minimize conflict through the convergence of the interests of the elderly with those of other "demanding" groups. Political constraints may dictate the abandonment of a universal NHI plan in the early 1980s; those within the gerontological community pressing for special programs may face the choice of continuing their demands or submerging them in support for broader, less adequate, benefit provisions.

More specific analysis of health insurance policy occurs against the background of the need for medical services, the extent to which those needs are presently met, and the general experiences of the population using those services. Data regarding health care utilization and expenditures by elderly Americans provide the context for analyzing the implications for the elderly of various forms of national health insurance.

While older people are comparatively less often afflicted with illnesses classified as "acute" (lasting less than three months), their associated disability and utilization of services are greater than those of younger persons. The elderly are much more likely than younger persons to suffer from one or more chronic conditions, to be limited in activity, and to use a physician's services. The elderly also have a substantially greater likelihood of being hospitalized and of being in the hospital longer for a given illness. And the elderly are clearly heavy users of institutional services such as nursing homes and personal care homes.

In 1977, although the elderly represented only 11 percent of the population, they accounted for 29 percent of personal health care expenditures. Sixty-seven percent of that bill for health services for the elderly was paid out of public funds, primarily Medicare and Medicaid (substantially more than for any other age group). Most of the remaining 27 percent of the total, an average of $613 per person, came directly from the resources of the elderly and their families. Such expenditures for health services are burdensome on the elderly, who are on average poorer than younger people. Moreover, the elderly individual's medical expenses and personal income tend to be inversely related.

ASSESSMENT OF THREE NHI PROPOSALS

Three health insurance proposals, each representing one of the three categories of proposals discussed above, can be assessed with regard to their implications for the elderly, taking into consideration the circumstances just discussed. These three proposals are:

1. The Long-Ribicoff-Waggoner bill
2. The Comprehensive Health Insurance Plan (CHIP)
3. The Kennedy-Corman plan

They will be evaluated on the basis of their eligibility provisions, coverage, financing, and administration.

Eligibility

The Kennedy-Corman plan can be ranked first on the basis of eligibility provisions affecting the elderly, since it has no income or age restrictions. CHIP ranks second, because it would continue Medicare coverage and improve Medicaid coverage for the poor elderly by setting national eligibility standards that would be higher than those in any state. The Long-Ribicoff-Waggoner proposal ranks third, because it would continue Medicare but would set national standards for Medicaid at a level higher than most, but not all, of the states.

Coverage

Assessment of the proposals on the basis of coverage is less straightforward. Because of the complexity of evaluating the proposals service by service, and because some of the data required for a full comparative assessment of the three proposals on the basis of service coverage cannot be specified until implementation, a firm ranking of the three proposals on this basis has not been attempted. It can be argued that the elderly require different forms of coverage than other groups and that assessment should be made on that basis. That is, some services—such as intermediate care and prescription drugs—must be covered, and coverage of services in general must be oriented toward chronic rather than acute conditions if health insurance is to best serve the most needy aged. However, if one assumes that the elderly benefit as much by general breadth of coverage as by coverage of specific services, it is significant that the Kennedy-Corman plan can be ranked highest and the

Long-Ribicoff-Waggoner plan lowest on comprehensiveness of coverage.

Financing

The elderly benefit to the extent that they do not make premium contributions or that premium contributions are graduated by income, and to the extent that they do not share costs or that cost sharing varies progressively by income up to set maximums. On these criteria, the Kennedy-Corman plan is the greatest improvement over the present system, because elderly beneficiaries would not contribute to its revenues except to the extent that they paid taxes, had unearned income, or were employed. CHIP ranks second, because premium and cost-sharing contributions by low-income, high-risk elderly persons would be graduated by income with specified maximums. The elderly would fare slightly better than they do presently under the Long-Ribicoff-Waggoner plan, primarily because of the limit placed on inpatient liability.

It should be noted that the financial implications for the elderly of cost-sharing provisions go beyond beneficiary payments themselves to the likelihood that the elderly, because of their substantial aversion to risk demonstrated in the Medicare program, will purchase supplemental first-dollar insurance coverage for which premiums exceed expected returns.

Administration

A fourth insurance system characteristic, administrative arrangements, has a particular significance for the elderly. Many of the aged are physically disabled or experience restricted mobility, and some are mentally impaired. They can better cope with health institutions when eligibility is determined on a few criteria and by one local agency, when eligibility is retained without period renewal, and when restrictions on insurance coverage are minimal and concise.

The Kennedy-Corman plan ranks first on simplicity of eligibility determination, with little distinction possible on this basis between the other two plans. While the plans vary in terms of restrictiveness of coverage, the fact that all have restrictions and limitations makes rankings on simplicity-of-coverage provisions difficult.

In general, then, the three NHI proposals reviewed here as examples of three categories of proposals—the Kennedy-Corman plan, CHIP, and the Long-Ribicoff-Waggoner plan—can be ranked first through third, respectively, in terms of their improvement on insurance coverage for the aged. By these same standards—eligibility range, services covered, financing, and administrative arrangements—it appears that the elderly would be better off under any of the major national health insurance proposals than they are now under Medicare and Medicaid. In such proposed plans, eligibility would be broader and less burdensome to establish, more services would be covered (except in states presently offering the most generous Medicaid coverage), services would be less oriented toward acute care, patient cost sharing would be reduced, and administration would be simplified (Davidson and Marmor 1980).

SOME NECESSARY CAUTIONS

The fact that NHI could help to equalize access to medical care for the elderly, as well as for all other Americans, has unquestionable social value. But two facts are often overlooked in our preoccupation with insurance issues.

The first is that insurance mechanisms can cause the unnecessary "medicalization" of services on the periphery of coverage, some of which are important services for the elderly. For example, the array of services that can be provided to the noninstitutionalized disabled ranges from the medical to the nonmedical, though the fact that there is a wide variety of medical rationales for services often does not permit a clean differentiation between the two types of service on a case-by-case basis. The medically oriented services are often categorized as "home health" or "personal care" services. Home health services are more likely than personal care services to be insured, but personal care services are presently insured, for example, under some Medicaid programs. Furthermore, the distinction between an individual's need for medical personal care services and nonmedical personal care services provided by social service agencies can be blurred.

National health insurance is likely to generate pressure to expand coverage to include personal care services as well as home health and, in turn, to create incentives for nonmedical personal care to become medically oriented. The cost implications of this type of coverage expansion for which the need can seem infinite are staggering, but equally significant is the attendant potential for changes in the nature of care delivered, the relationship between recipient and provider, and the institutions involved.

The second fact that is widely acknowledged but still not truly taken into account in the deliberations on national health insurance is that increased medical care is not analogous to improved health. The elderly's pursuit of health must go beyond support for NHI to compelling society's attention to their basic economic security, their role in the workplace, and the implications of evolving family structures. To the extent that financing of medical care preempts support of other social programs, the overall welfare of the elderly may suffer. And the risk of this happening, if indeed it has not already begun, is real.

It is important that these issues not be neglected in the continuing debate over national health insurance for Americans; it seems quite clear, however, that whatever style program is eventually adopted will have important implications for all Americans, not just the elderly.

APPENDIX A
HISTORY OF NATIONAL HEALTH
INSURANCE IN THE UNITED STATES

National health insurance has been an issue in American politics since 1912, when Teddy Roosevelt supported it in his campaign for president under the Progressive party banner. Although Roosevelt and the Progressive party were defeated, support for national health insurance did not die. For nearly a decade, the American Association for Labor Legislation

(AALL) continued to fight for national health insurance legislation, though by 1920, when the American Medical Association withdrew its support and antireform sentiment prevailed in the nation, it was clear that the efforts of the AALL were doomed to failure. National health insurance again appeared on the political landscape during the Great Depression, but it was one of the few reforms proposed in the New Deal era that met defeat. The Truman administration's efforts to secure passage of a national health insurance program during the late 1940s and early 1950s were also unsuccessful. In the 1960s, public attention was again focused on the issue. Congress took a limited step in the direction of national health insurance in 1965 when it enacted the Medicare and Medicaid programs, which provided publicly supported health care for the aged (see The Urban Institute 1979).

APPENDIX B
SELECTED NATIONAL HEALTH
INSURANCE PROPOSALS: BRIEF
SKETCHES

Catastrophic Health Insurance and Medical
Reform Act (Long-Ribicoff Bill, S. 350)

General Approach The plan includes three components:

1. A catastrophic illness insurance program for the general population provided through a federally administered plan or through approved private plans.
2. A federal medical assistance program for the poor and the medically needy.
3. Provisions for federal certification of qualified private basic health insurance.

Benefits Under both the federal and private catastrophic plans, individuals would be covered for the following after they had spent 60 days in the hospital: additional days in the hospital, up to 100 days in a skilled nursing facility, and home health services. After a family had spent $2,000 on medical expenses, it would be covered for physician services, laboratory and x-ray services, and medical supplies and appliances.

Under the medical assistance program, beneficiaries would be fully covered for hospital services and stays in skilled nursing and intermediate care facilities; they would be charged three dollars per visit for their first ten physician visits, with full coverage thereafter; and they would be fully covered for laboratory and x-ray services, family-planning services, maternity care, and children's medical examinations.

Administration   The federal catastrophic coverage plan would be administered by the federal government through fiscal agents, except for employers who prefer to purchase coverage from approved private insurance plans. The medical assistance plan would be administered by the federal government through fiscal agents.

Provider Reimbursement   Under the federally administered catastrophic coverage plan, physicians would be reimbursed on a fee-for-service basis according to usual, customary, and reasonable (UCR) charge screens. Physicians could charge fees above the government rate. Hospitals would be reimbursed for the "reasonable costs" of care. Under private catastrophic coverage plans, reimbursement methods would be determined by individual insurance carriers.

Under the medical assistance plan, physicians would be reimbursed on a fee-for-service basis according to UCR charge screens, but they would be required to accept the plan's payment as payment in full. Hospitals would be reimbursed for the "reasonable costs" of care.

Financing   The federal catastrophic coverage plan would be financed through a 1 percent payroll tax on employers, who would be allowed a federal income tax credit equal to 50 percent of the tax. Employers offering private plans would also be subject to the 1 percent payroll tax, but the tax would be reduced by the actuarial value of their private coverage.

Federal and state general revenues would be used to finance the medical assistance plan. State shares would be fixed annual amounts based on state Medicaid costs for the types of services provided under the new program, with some adjustments for continued expenditures on services not covered by the program.

Health Care for All Americans Act (Kennedy-Waxman Bill, H.R. 5191)

General Approach   Comprehensive health-care benefits would be provided to all U.S. citizens and legal resident aliens by mandating their enrollment in a private insurance plan, either through an employer or on an individual basis. Premiums would vary with income, and government would pay in full for the poor. Premiums and payments to providers would be negotiated within a predetermined national health insurance budget.

Benefits   The plan would cover hospital inpatient and outpatient services (limits on services for mental illness); up to 100 days of care in a skilled nursing facility following hospitalization of 3 days or more; physician visits (limits on services for mental conditions); up to 100 home health visits per year; other medical and health services, including x-ray and laboratory services, medical equipment, and prostheses; outpatient drugs for Medicare patients for the treatment of chronic illness; outpatient physical, speech, and occupational therapy; 2 days of mental health day-care services for each day of allowed inpatient psychiatric benefits; and one audiological exam per year and one hearing aid every three years.

Administration   The federal government, through the program's newly established National Health Board, would set national policy guidelines and oversee implementation, compute national and state health insurance budgets, and set rules for paying for services within budgets. State governments would nominate members to State Health Boards, which would negotiate prospective budgets and fee schedules for provider payment, oversee insurance enrollment, and guarantee provider payment. State governments would administer residual Medicaid programs. Private insurers and health maintenance organizations would establish national consortia to collect and distribute premiums and participate in provider payment negotiations. Individual plans would enroll members and pay providers.

Provider Reimbursement   Hospitals, home health agencies, neighborhood health and other health centers, and skilled nursing facilities would be reimbursed based on prospectively set rates consistent with approved budgets. Physicians would be reimbursed according to fee schedules subject to overall budget limits. Health maintenance organizations would be reimbursed through capitation payments (fixed amounts per patient per year regardless of the number of services provided).

Financing   The program would have seven major sources of financing: (1) wage-related premiums and (2) premiums on substantial amounts of nonwage income (premiums would be calculated as a percentage of income); (3) state payments on behalf of AFDC beneficiaries and state institutional populations; (4) federal payments on behalf of SSI beneficiaries and federal institutional populations; (5) voluntary payments on behalf of U.S. residents employed by foreign governments or international organizations; (6) Medicare taxes and premiums; and (7) general revenues.

National Health Plan (Phase I) (Carter Administration Proposal, S. 1812)

General Approach   The plan includes two components:

1.   Healthcare, a public plan providing comprehensive coverage to the aged, the disabled, the poor, and the near-poor and offering catastrophic, prenatal, delivery, and infant care coverage to individuals and firms who have difficulty obtaining such insurance in the private sector.
2.   Employer-Guaranteed Coverage, a program requiring employers to provide all full-time employees, their spouses, and dependent children with health benefits meeting uni-

form federal standards. Employers would be required to pay at least 75 percent of the health insurance premium.

Benefits Benefits under Healthcare and Employer-Guaranteed Coverage would include hospital care; up to 100 days per year in a skilled nursing facility; up to 20 days per year in a mental hospital; physician services; diagnostic services; up to 200 home health visits per year; up to $1,000 per year in outpatient mental health care; medical equipment; laboratory and x-ray services; prenatal care; delivery; preventive and acute child health care in the first year of life; family-planning services; and immunizations.

The following would be eligible for coverage under Healthcare: all persons now eligible for Medicare plus any person over age sixty-five whose income is less than 55 percent of the federal poverty standard; all persons now eligible for cash assistance and others whose income is less than 55 percent of the federal poverty standard; any applicant for prenatal, delivery, and infant care coverage; any person whose medical expenses cause a "spend down" to 55 percent of the federal poverty standard; and any other person or group who pays a specified premium (coverage subject to a $2,500 deductible).

All full-time employees, their spouses, and dependent children would be eligible for Employer-Guaranteed Coverage. Beneficiaries would be subject to a maximum deductible of $2,500. After the deductible had been met, plans would be required to provide all benefits available under Healthcare and could offer broader coverage. There would be no cost sharing on prenatal services, delivery, and infant care.

Administration The federal government would administer Healthcare through fiscal agents and would regulate private plans. Private insurers would underwrite and sell plans for most current beneficiaries and add new beneficiaries under Employer-Guaranteed Coverage.

Provider Reimbursement Under Healthcare, hospitals would be reimbursed for the "reasonable costs" of care but, under both Healthcare and Employer-Guaranteed Coverage, reimbursement would be limited according to provisions of hospital cost-containment legislation (separately introduced). Physicians providing services to Healthcare patients would be reimbursed according to a fee schedule. All physicians accepting Healthcare patients would be required to accept the fee schedule amount as payment in full. After the first year of implementation, the fee schedule would be revised through negotiations between Healthcare and physician representatives. There would be no restrictions on physician payments under Employer-Guaranteed Coverage.

Financing   Healthcare would be financed with the hospital insurance portion of the Social Security tax, premiums paid by nonpoor aged and disabled enrollees (equivalent to Medicare Part B premiums), and state and federal general revenues. Employer-Guaranteed Coverage would be financed with premiums paid by individuals (up to 25 percent) and employers (at least 75 percent).

Consumer Choice Health Plan (Developed by Alain Enthoven for Joseph A. Califano, Jr., Former Secretary of Health, Education, and Welfare, September 1977)

General Approach   All legal U.S. residents, except those eligible for Medicare, would receive tax credits based on income and actuarial risk categories for a proportion of premiums paid for private health insurance plans. The poor would receive vouchers covering the full cost of premiums.

Benefits   To qualify for tax credits, private insurance plans would be required to provide a basic minimum benefit package (oriented toward protection against catastrophic costs) and to specify maximum individual or family out-of-pocket outlays for a one- or two-year period. The dollar amount of the maximum and benefits beyond the minimum would be set by the individual plans. Health maintenance organizations, as well as traditional insurance plans, would participate. All plans would be required to set community rates, participate in periodic government-run open enrollment, and offer a low-option plan limited to the basic benefits defined by law. Medicare benefits would be expanded to conform to benefits for the rest of the population. The 150-day limit on hospital days would be removed, and an annual limit on out-of-pocket expenses would be set.

Administration   The program could be administered by the federal government or jointly by the federal government and the states. Tax credits would be administered through the Internal Revenue Service, and vouchers for the poor would be administered through a reformed cash assistance system that would be almost entirely federal. Plan qualifications and enrollment could be handled by either the federal government or state governments.

Provider Reimbursement   No method is specified; reimbursement could be left to private insurers' discretion or subject to government regulation.

Financing   The plan would be financed primarily with federal general revenues, perhaps with some contribution from state and individual premiums beyond the tax credit.

Source: The Urban Institute. 1979. *Policy and Research Report* 9, no. 2 (Winter):6–8. Reprinted with permission of The Urban Institute, publisher.

REFERENCES

Binstock, R. 1979. "A Policy Agenda on Aging for the 1980s." *National Journal* 11: 1711–17.

Davidson, S., and T.R. Marmor. 1980. *The Cost of Living Longer: National Health Insurance and the Elderly*. Lexington, Mass.: Lexington Books.

Enthoven, Alain. 1980. *Health Plan*. Reading, Massachusetts: Addison-Wesley.

Feder, J.; J. Holahan; and T.R. Marmor. 1980. *National Health Insurance: Conflicting Goals and Policy Choices*. Washington, D.C.: The Urban Institute.

Marmor, T.R.; B. Gold; and E. Kutza. 1976. "United States Social Policy on Old Age: Present Patterns and Predictions." In *Social*

Policy, Social Ethics, and the Aging Society, edited by B. Neugarten and C. Havighurst, pp. 9–21. Washington, D.C.: Government Printing Office.

*Report of the President's Commission for a National Agenda for the
Eighties.* 1980. Washington, D.C.: Government Printing Office.

The Urban Institute. 1979. *Policy and Research Report* 9, no. 2
(Winter).

U.S. Office of Management and Budget. 1979. Executive Office of the
President, Special Analysis L., "Health." In *Special Analyses,
Budget of the United States Government, Fiscal Year 1979.* Wash-
ington, D.C.: Government Printing Office.

2 PROSPECTS FOR INCREASING HUMAN LONGEVITY

Leonard Hayflick

Despite all the conflicting views on the causes of biological aging, most gerontologists agree that, after reaching sexual maturity, individuals in most species accumulate physiological decrements that increase their likelihood of dying. In fact, for humans, the data, first analyzed by the English actuary Gompertz in 1825, reveal that the force of mortality doubles every seven years beyond the age of thirty—that is, after maturity, the rate and probability of dying are exponential with increasing age. Although subject to some individual variation, a variety of human physiological functions show a slow, nearly linear decline from thirty years of age. The rate constants for this linear loss seem to occur at about 0.8 to 0.9 percent loss per year of the functional capacity present at the age of thirty.

The common impression that the triumphs of modern medicine have lengthened the human life span is not supported by either vital statistics or biological evidence. The fact is that in the developed countries, the prevention and treatment of those ills that occur in the early years have improved; consequently, more people are reaching what appears to be an immutable upper age limit. Thus, life expectancy has increased (Figure 2–1), but the human life span has remained virtually unchanged since recorded history. Medical achievements have simply al-

Figure 2–1. Average Length of Life From Ancient to Modern Times

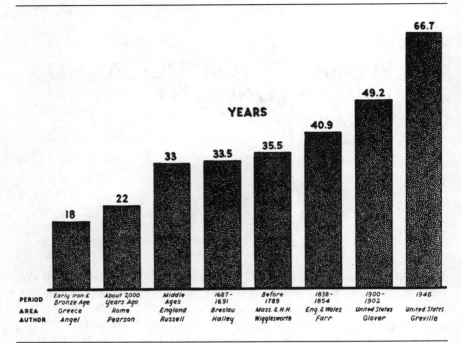

	Early Iron & Bronze Age	About 2,000 Years Ago	Middle Ages	1687– 1691	Before 1789	1838– 1854	1900– 1902	1946
PERIOD								
AREA	Greece	Rome	England	Breslau	Mass. & N.H.	Eng. & Wales	United States	United States
AUTHOR	Angel	Pearson	Russell	Halley	Wigglesworth	Farr	Glover	Greville

lowed more persons to reach the limit of what appears to be a fixed life span. Deaths in the early years are becoming increasingly less frequent in the developed countries, resulting in life tables that are simply becoming more rectangular, indicated by the direction of the arrow in Figure 2–2. In many privileged countries, one now can expect to become reasonably old, which is a relatively new phenomenon.

EFFECTS OF THE RESOLUTION OF DISEASES

If the two leading causes of death in the United States—heart disease and stroke—are successfully eliminated, approximately twelve years of additional life can be expected. If the third greatest cause of death—cancer—is eliminated, about two years of additional life expectancy will result. The net increase at birth in life expectancy achieved in the United States from 1900 to 1950 was almost twenty years. This increase resulted from a decline in the large number of deaths that occurred before the age of sixty-five. On the other hand, the gain in life expectancy at sixty-five and seventy-five years of age from 1900 to 1969 was, respectively, only 2.9 and 2.2 years.

What would be the effect on human longevity and the human life span in a world in which all causes of death resulting from disease and accidents were totally eliminated? The effect on human longevity would be to realize the ultimate rectangular curve (see Figure 2–2) in which citizens would live out their lives free of the fear of premature death, but with the certain fate that their normal physiological decrements would result in death on about their hundredth birthday.

These concepts have forced gerontologists to the conclusion that the disease-oriented approach to medical research might increase life expectancy but will have little impact on increasing the human life span. If such an increase is desirable—and

Figure 2–2.   Life Tables

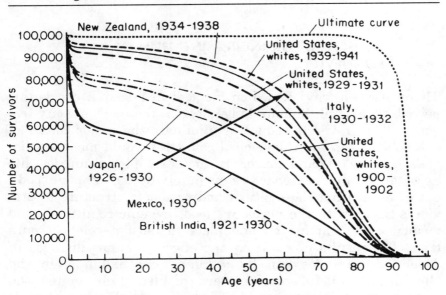

Source: Adapted from Comfort, A., 1964, *Ageing: The Biology of Senescence,* Reprinted by permission of Routledge and Kegan Paul, Ltd.

there is considerable doubt that it is—one must first separate the disease-related causes of death from the age-dependent normal physiological decrements that give rise to manifestations of old age. The diseases of old age are simply superimposed on these normal physiological decrements, but must be separately regarded if one is rationally to consider increasing the human life span. Although age-associated physiological decrements surely increase vulnerability to disease, the fundamental causes of death are not diseases but the physiological decrements that make their occurrence more likely.

Biomedical research has trained its heavy artillery almost exclusively on the disease-associated causes of death. Scant attention has been paid to the underlying causes of biological aging that are not disease associated but which, in clocklike fashion, dictate for each species a specific maximum life span. To be sure, the physiological decrements that occur in advancing years increase vulnerability to disease, but unless more attention is paid to the fundamental non-disease-related biological causes of aging, the fate of each person will be death on about the hundredth birthday.

PROSPECTS FOR INCREASING HUMAN LONGEVITY

There are two ways in which biomedical research can be expected to extend human longevity in the next twenty-five years. The first is to reduce or eliminate the major causes of death, which in most developed countries would mean cardiovascular diseases and cancer. In the developing countries, life expectancy can be extended immediately by the simple expedient of motivating the political and economic structure to provide citizens with the necessary food, hygenic conditions, and medical care that are commonplace in most developed countries. The results of reducing the effect of minor diseases in developed countries will be minimal. For example, in the United States, if tuberculosis were completely eliminated, the gain in life expectancy would be less than a 0.05 year. Thus, it could be argued that if an increase in life expectation becomes the main goal of biomedical research in the developed countries, all such research should be directed toward the elimination of the two major causes of death. This position, although less than humane and not likely to attract many adherents, is nonetheless the most logical conclusion to be derived from life-table studies and the projections.

The second way in which biomedical research can deal with human longevity is to address itself specifically to the underlying non-disease-related fundamental biological causes of age changes. These are not regarded as diseases but are the basic biological changes that result in physiological decrements characteristic of aging. On these changes is superimposed an increasing vulnerability to disease. Such an approach, then, does not directly concern itself with efforts to increase human life expectancy, but rather to extend what appears to be a fixed life span that differs in its length for humans and all other animal species.

As a measure of the current effort put forth toward these two approaches, funds spent in the United States on cardiovascular disease and cancer research are about twenty-five times greater than the funds spent in gerontology. It is also probable that in both these areas the number of researchers, and consequently the amount of effort, also differs twenty-five-fold. Consequently, the likelihood that any significant increase in human longevity will occur in the next quarter-century depends on either (1) significantly better cure rates for cardiovascular diseases and cancer; or (2) significant advances in our understanding and ability to manipulate the biological clocks that set for each species a mean maximum life span.

If potential success in either of these endeavors can be measured by the current attitudes and priorities of the biomedical research establishment in the United States, then clearly the search for cardiovascular disease and cancer cures is much more likely to effect human longevity than is gerontological research. A further conclusion is that by curing these two diseases, a maximum of fourteen years of additional life expectancy could be attained, but with successful efforts to increase the life span itself, no fixed end point is ruled out. Furthermore, the resolution of the two leading killers will in no way reverse or halt the decline in physiological decrements characteristic of age changes, whereas efforts to increase the life span could lead to such a reversal. Clearly, research in cardiovascular diseases and cancer should not be stopped, but if our goal is to maximize opportunities to effectively increase human longevity, then our current priorities are seriously out of balance. If this imbalance continues unchanged, the likelihood is extremely small indeed that the research accomplishments of a handful of underfunded gerontologists will affect the human life span.

DEMOGRAPHIC PROJECTIONS

It is well known that in the developed countries the proportion of persons over the age of sixty-five has been steadily increasing. In the last one hundred years, their proportions within the total population in the United States have increased from 3 to 10 percent, and the aged have become a larger proportion of the nonworking component of the population, including nonworking youth. This nonworking population component is largely supported by the workforce itself, and if current population trends continue, the elderly will command increasingly more support.

Within forty years those over sixty-five are expected to number nearly 400 million in the United States (see Figure 2–3). This prediction does not take into account any major resolution within forty years of the two leading causes of death, cardiovascular disease and cancer. If some significant cure rate were to occur, however, the United States might have as many persons over sixty-five as under fifteen in the year 2025.

If zero population growth were to be achieved and maintained in the United States, the family size of old persons would obviously be reduced, and along with that reduction would come a diminution in the economic, social, and psychological benefits that now accrue from adult children. The inevitable consequence would be a further acceleration of current trends, in which governments would provide more health care, food, housing, recreation, and income to the elderly.

Since zero population might be achieved in a number of countries by the year 2025, it is interesting to speculate on the consequences of another extreme condition—a population in

Figure 2–3.   Growth of the Population 65 Years and Over: 1900 to 2020

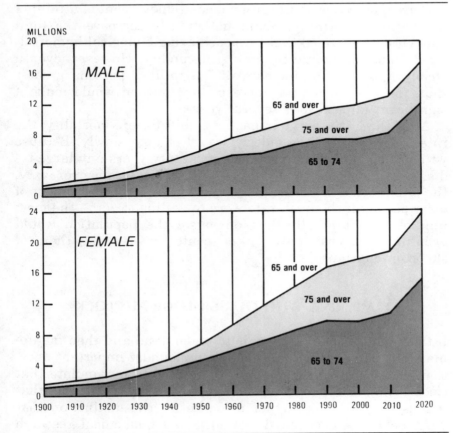

which no one dies at all. The immediate effect on the growth rate of the total population would be significant, since the growth rate would be increased by the amount of the current death rate. In the long run, however, the increase would not be dramatic (see Siegel 1976). The increase in growth rate would be somewhat less than 0.5 million persons per year in the United States population of 250 million—that is, over and above the number of births now being added to the population each year. (In 1974, the number of births was approximately 3 million. With no mortality, the number of births would be an additional 0.5 million, based on the projection that those women who now die in childhood would survive and would bear children.)

Consequently, even the stupendous achievement of attaining biological immortality would not greatly increase the total population—provided that those achieving biological immortality did not concomitantly gain in fecundity. However, even a steady-state annual increase of 0.5 million persons greater than the present annual increase of 3 million would make a significant impact after several years.

After the initial large impact of a shift to zero mortality, the rate of increase of the elderly would change slowly. Because with the current life expectancy of seventy years any large reductions in death rates would be limited to persons over sixty, the elimination of all deaths would increase the proportion of older people. If the birth rate were to decline to zero—the most unlikely event of all—then obviously the population would eventually consist entirely of centenarians and then of supercentenarians.

TAMPERING WITH OUR BIOLOGICAL CLOCK

If the goal of biogerontology is to understand and then manipulate our biological clock, then one profoundly important question arises: How desirable is it to be able to manipulate that clock? The answer to this question is not simple. The fact that it must be asked is further evidence for the distinction that must be made between disease-oriented biomedical research and gerontological research. The goals of gerontological research are distinct from other biomedical goals because we are not certain whether the resolution of the physiological decrements of old age will indeed benefit the individual or society as a whole.

There are many possible scenarios that might result from the control of age changes, and each has an important negative side effect. Take, for example, the possibility that biomedical research might result in the total elimination of all causes of death. If this were achieved and no control were had on the biological clock itself, the result might be a society whose members would live full, physically vigorous, youthful lives until the ninth decade when the physiological decrements of old age would lead to sudden death.

If, on the other hand, biogerontologists were to learn how to tamper with our biological clock, to what end would one choose to reset this clock? Surely one wouldn't choose to spend an additional ten years suffering from the infirmities of old age—yet that might, initially, be the only way to intervene. Is society prepared to cope with individuals whose only choice might be between naturally occurring death and ten or more years spent with the viscissitudes of old age? We can hardly deal with a maximum life span of, say, ninety years, to say nothing of the further social, economic, and political dislocations that might occur if we add a decade to this figure.

Aside from this possibility, it is also worth considering the prospect of clock tampering in which we could spend more years at a particular developmental stage of our lives than we now do. The clock might be stalled for ten years at, for example, the chronological age of twenty. But is this desirable? Probably most of us would decide that the time during which we would like our biological clocks arrested should correspond to those years in which maximum life satisfaction and productivity occurred. Yet if we were forced to make such a decision, it would probably have to be made prospectively. Even more complex is the question of when in the human life span individuals are most productive, and life satisfaction greatest. An exhaustive study of this question was made by Harvey C. Lehman in *Age and Achievement* (1953). The conclusion to be reached from this data is that, depending on the particular area of human endeavor, the time of maximum productivity can occur anywhere throughout the human life span. Thus clock tampering becomes a game that very few of us are capable of playing.

GOALS FOR BIOGERONTOLOGY

Having presented here only a few of the possible goals of biological research in aging, it should be clear that a simple decision cannot be made. Although it is simple to state and conceptually easy to understand, I have purposely avoided the

notion of biological immortality. I have done this for one principle reason: to attain it is so far beyond any practical realization that any discussion of it would be more science fiction
than likely science fact.

Furthermore, among the most serious effects of even a modest success by biological gerontologists in increasing human
life expectancy are the societal consequences. Most gerontological sociologists are persuaded that even as little as a five-year
increase in life expectancy at, say, age seventy-five would be so
profound as to rupture our present economic, medical, and welfare institutions.

In spite of the apparent dilemma in stating goals for gerontological research, there is, I believe, one goal that appears to
be wholly desirable and even attainable as a short-range objective. That would simply be to reduce the physiological decrements associated with biological aging so that vigorous,
productive, nondependent lives would be led up until the maximum life span. Implicit in this notion is that the quality of life
is more important than its quantity.

The goal of gerontological research in the future should be
to understand the biological basis of aging in order to extend
the number of vigorous and productive years, and to reduce the
time spent in senility and the infirmities of old age. Of what
value is immortality, if by achieving it one extends the infirmities? Two modern versions of this theme exist in Aldous
Huxley's *After Many a Summer Dies the Swan* and Oscar
Wilde's *Picture of Dorian Gray*. In fact, the Gerontological Society itself has as its motto a similar concept: "To add life to
years, not just years to life." I would therefore challenge the
view that the goal of research in aging is simply to increase
longevity.

If longevity is to be increased merely by extending the years
of our infirmities, then the goal is not worth seeking. This indeed is the modern dilemma faced by many physicians who are
using every means for prolonging the terminal stages of disease in the name of prolonging life at the expense of continuing the agony of certain death. The goal that appears to be not
only more desirable but indeed more attainable is not the extension of longevity per se, but the extension of our most vigorous and productive years. If tampering with our biological

clock ever becomes a reality, I believe that it would be tragic in the extreme if such procedures were to result only in the extension of those years spent in declining physical and mental health. Having said this, what are the prospects of achieving increased longevity?

SOME IMMEDIATE POSSIBILITIES

Among all the areas of human health care, there is probably no other arena of greater quackery than the legion of alleged life-extending nostrums, diets, exercises, injections, and other procedures foisted on a gullible public. Most gerontologists agree that none of these claims have been authenticated by scientific proof.

There is, in the judgment of some gerontologists, at least one comparatively innocuous way in which the human life span probably might be extended significantly. The method is based on classic studies made by Clive McKay in the 1930s and since confirmed in many laboratories for a number of animal species, including rats, in which it was first described. The method is simply to reduce the caloric intake to such a level that undernutrition, but no malnutrition, occurs. This is done by providing an animal with a diet sufficient in all necessary nutrients, but very low in calories. Longevity can then be increased by as much as 50 percent. The effects are most pronounced if caloric-restriction diets are initiated when animals are very young. This results in a stretching out of the developmental stages so that infancy, puberty, maturity, adulthood, and aging simply occur at later-than-usual points in time, thereby increasing the total life span.

On the assumption that undernutrition in humans would yield similar results, it is of interest to observe that in the forty years since this has been known, no human has consciously chosen to do it, even the biologists who know the data best. Considering the number of nostrums and treatments that have been foisted on a gullible public as antiaging regimens, this lack of interest in underfeeding is, on superficial consideration, remarkable. On the supposition that the method is widely known, that it works, and that it is not dangerous, the main conclusion that can be drawn from the notable lack of interest is that for most people the quality of life is more important than its quantity. If this is so, then an important lesson can be learned. Any method that might increase human longevity is unacceptable if it affects, even minimally, the enjoyment of life.

TO SLEEP, PERCHANCE TO DREAM

There remains yet another method for increasing life expectancy that bears consideration. Although it will not result in an extension of life on an absolute time scale, it is interesting to consider a form of increased longevity based on the self-evident supposition that life can be lived only when individuals are both physically and mentally active. Since, for most individuals, sleep consumes nearly one-third of our lives, a reduction in the time spent sleeping should result in an increase in productive occupation and the enjoyment of life—that is, if sleep itself is not considered to be either productive or enjoyable. Sleep researchers tell us that no detectable negative effect on health has been observed in those individuals who have learned how to make a modest reduction in the length of time usually spent asleep. The impact of this change would be profound, for if we were to reduce by one-half hour the average of eight hours spent sleeping, the net effect on life extension would be an increase of more than two years. This increase in life expectancy is equivalent to living in a society where cancer deaths have been totally eliminated. Instead of any biological advances resulting in the prolongation of human life, this scenario could result from a social movement of an organization of "Awakists" whose members learned to do with less sleep in order to gain the additional time that might be productively and happily spent.

REDUCED METABOLIC RATES

Another similar approach to "prolongevity" would be to mimic in humans the reduced metabolism of those animals who pass the winter in hibernation or the summer in estivation. The value of this method presupposes that a slowing of metabolic rates for prolonged periods of time could, in the long run, extend the life span. Although no compelling evidence exists that a reduced metabolic rate might extend the human life span, this approach has some merit in its likely feasibility, since the state could probably be induced by drugs or by cold treatment, producing a controlled inhibition of the sympathetic nervous system and a twilight sleep resembling narcosis.

Assuming that this were feasible, significant questions of ethics and societal consequences of such an action must be considered. If it were possible to reduce the metabolic rate in humans over a span of, say, ten years, with the result that five more years would be added to the life span, would this be useful? What ten-year period of hibernation would a subject choose in order to effect a gain in years at some future time? One might choose to arrest oneself in a sleeplike trance for perhaps ten years, beginning at the age of forty, with instructions to be awakened in a decade so as to enjoy ten more years with one's grandchildren as young adults rather than as infants.

The potential societal dislocations resulting from such a scenario are awesome. Family councils might have to be held in order to determine who should be allowed to hibernate, when, and for how long, so as to avoid father being awakened at a biological age of forty only to celebrate mother's eightieth birthday. Other variations on these kinds of asynchronous scenarios can lead to amusing solutions of current problems. Consider our society's negative attitude toward May-December marriages. The older partner might hibernate for a few decades in order to allow the younger partner to either grow up or catch up.

CHANGING ATTITUDES

It is sometimes observed that there are no gerontologists—just biochemists, cell biologists, and immunologists working in gerontology. Many serious biologists with an interest in aging still hold at arm's length the appellation "gerontologists." Some think that the problem is simply too complex seriously to believe that it will yield to experimentation; others contend that the many pseudoscientific fringe groups still in search of biological immortality have had such a pervasive influence on the field that to formally associate oneself with it would be to suffer an unseemly stigma.

Happily these convictions have become less tenable in the past few years, and a significant change in attitude toward the science of gerontology has occurred. A realization is now developing that biological aging is no more complex than are problems in embryology, development, neurobiology, cancer research, or genetics. It is no longer possible to contend that efforts by gerontologists to reverse the aging process are akin to medieval alchemy, in view of the fact that all successful biomedical research has the net effect of prolonging life. Thus there is no rational reason to discourage research on the fundamental causes of age changes. Established gerontologists are no longer apologetically explaining their interest in aging, and young scientists are beginning to appreciate that the fundamental problems are less intractable than their predecessors thought. Public awareness of this neglected field has, commendably, resulted in sufficient recognition that an Institute on Aging has finally been created within the National Institutes of Health.

For the first time, the discipline of gerontology has been given enough national recognition at the biomedical level to make real the possibility that meaningful efforts will be made to understand the biology of aging. The field now has a level of visibility almost compatible with the magnitude of the problem. Even more important is the implied notion that something can and should be done about biological age changes. The period of utter disregard of the field has now passed, and recognition that the problem is not intractable has finally been established.

Although the goals of research into the biology of aging may well be as clouded ten years from now as they are today, it is still a virtual certainty that research in the field will continue. Until the objectives are better defined, however, the fallibility of those of us engaged in gerontological research makes it unlikely that a full understanding of the aging process will be revealed soon.

Since the discipline of biogerontology will continue to flourish even in the absence of clearly delineated goals, what are the most likely research trails leading to a better understanding of aging? It seems clear that the trail will take us into the cell and terminate with a full understanding of information-containing molecules (see Hayflick 1975, 1976, 1980a, 1980b).

THE FUTURE OF AGING RESEARCH

The future of aging research is really a function of the quality and quantity of young investigators who are encouraged to enter this field. Biogerontology has long been regarded as an impractical pseudoscience dealt with only by eccentrics and charlatans. Research on aging has been neglected by qualified scientists, who perceive the field to be lacking in scientific respectability—a view doubtless encouraged by the fact that no area of biology has been more deceptive to the gullible or more profitable to the unscrupulous.

As a consequence of these considerations biogerontology has, until recently, attracted few scientists willing to risk their reputation by working in a field that suffered such a stigma. The notion that the biology of senescence is too complex to yield to experimentation is a myth. How much more complex is it than developmental biology? When the continuum of life is perceived from conception, biologists call it developmental biology; when perceived from its terminus, it is called gerontology. And if we can presume that a full understanding of the biology of development is possible, is it any less likely that the processes of aging can be understood?

REFERENCES

Hayflick, L. 1975. "Current Theories of Biological Aging." *Federation Proceedings.* 34:9–13.
Hayflick, L. 1976. "Biology of Aging." *New England Journal of Medicine* 295:1302–8.

Hayflick, L. 1980a. "Cell Aging." In *Annual Review of Gerontology and Geriatrics,* vol. 1, edited by C. Eisdorfer, pp. 26–67. New York: Springer Publishing Co.

Hayflick, L. 1980b. "The Cell Biology of Human Aging." *Scientific American* 242 (January): 158–66.

Lehman, H.C. 1953. *Age and Achievement.* Princeton: Princeton University Press.

McCay, C.M.; F. Pop; and W. Lunsford. 1956. "Experimental Prolongation of the Life Span." *Bulletin of the New York Academy of Medicine* 32:91–101.

Siegel, J.S. 1976. "Demographic Aspects of Aging and the Older Population in the United States." *Current Population Reports, Special Studies.* Series P-23, No. 59. Washington, D.C.: Government Printing Office.

Strehler, B.L., and A.S. Mildvan. 1960. "General Theory of Mortality and Aging." *Science* 132:14–21.

3 AGE AND THE LAW

George J. Alexander

> *Grow old along with me!*
> *The best is yet to be,*
> *The last of life for which the first was made.*
> Robert Browning, *Rabbi Ben Ezra*

Browning was a hopeless romantic. Huxley was more accurate when in *Brave New World* (1946) he had society cheerfully carting off the old to the neighborhood crematorium. As a practical matter, the old are a minority group, probably the least militant minority group in the country, although they have more to be militant about than many others. Their superior claim to being disgruntled is related to their entry into the group. For most minority group members, entry is both instantaneous and permanent. One is born black, Chicano, illegitimate; whatever societal disadvantage is visited on those minorities arrives early and is continuous. The hope for escape is virtually nonexistent. Indeed, a useful way of defining a minority group in need of special legal protection is by examining the immutability of its membership: the more immutable, the more the need for protection. Old people, however, come by their second-class status late in life, and it is at once more shocking and more terrible because it is unaccustomed.

45

So great is the fear of aging in this youth culture that psychological barriers are created against the recognition that we grow old. As packing the dying off to hospitals allows others to avoid a recognition of their own mortality, so thinking of the old as "them" sustains an illusion of eternal youth. The unfortunate result of this self-delusion, however, is a basic rejection of those excluded.

But the youth focus is not entirely to blame for the social mistreatment that accelerates with age. Two other catastrophic events play a major part. The first is a conjunction of galloping inflation and accelerated taxation of income and inheritance. Those forces together guarantee that most people will have to live from income rather than from their own savings, let alone the savings of prior generations. Yet income is routinely diminished as age increases.

The second event, of equal importance, is the shrinkage of the family. While in other societies the extended cohabiting family may range through several generations, in our culture one does not live with parents much beyond puberty. Cut off from income by loss of employment, taxed and inflated out of the value of their savings, with children whose autonomy demands that they approach even the institution of marriage with great suspicion, the old are simply catapulted into another world.

That world, familiar to other disadvantaged groups, is one of poverty, food stamps obtained after filling out voluminous questionnaires, welfare payments given out in endless lines and on rude conditions, obtrusive social workers, and often institutionalization. It is the managed society. It is a realm in which self-determination and autonomy in personal affairs—values otherwise highly prized by our society—are subordinated to the fulfillment of basic needs. The paternalism and benevolence of others may directly or indirectly force the older person to sacrifice freedom of choice in such personally significant areas as health care, in order to obtain a modicum of necessary services, even though the services actually provided are often quite inappropriate to the older person's needs.

As one can in time become accustomed to virtually any societal conditions—there is in fact a generation of governmentally created welfare clients—one can expect to find a number of people who have learned to live with and appreciate the security of being public charges. Some merely continue this status through old age. Most of the old, however—the *nouveau pauvre*—lack this "education." For them it is the first time in a food-stamp line, the first time on welfare, the first time in a public institution. Most old persons join the managed state only after a lifetime of freedom.

To a very limited extent, the law prohibits age discrimination. To a great extent, however, it approves and even requires disadvantage for the elderly. Legal prohibitions against age discrimination are easily stated. State statutes vary considerably, but federal legislation has principally taken three forms: the Age Discrimination in Employment Act of 1967, the Age Discrimination Act of 1975, and the Equal Credit Opportunity Act Amendment of 1976. The first outlaws compulsory retirement because of age under limited circumstances. The second act prohibits age-based discrimination in federally funded programs. Both acts leave a great deal to be desired. The present form of the Age Discrimination in Employment Act generally prohibits discharge based on age for employees between the ages of forty and seventy. It is certainly preferable to its predecessor version, which prohibited similar discrimination against those between forty and sixty-five. While that act did not require compulsory retirement at age sixty-five, it certainly went far toward legitimizing it. The present act has extended the age to seventy in the private sector, and has eliminated compulsory retirement because of age altogether in most federal service.

The Age Discrimination Act prohibits discrimination on the basis of age generally, but specifically exempts the use of age as a criterion for adverse treatment when such a criterion is used as a surrogate to measure some significant employee capacity. The act specifically allows age to be used, however, when it is a factor "necessary to the normal operation" of a program. Disparate treatment is also permissible if based on "reasonable factors other than age." Furthermore, despite legislative history stressing protection of the elderly, the act as interpreted applies equally to both young and old. Consequently, beneficial effects for the elderly are tempered by concern lest comparable rights be required for the very young. It is a concern very reminiscent of the Bakke-Weber conflicts that test the extent to which majoritarian rights must keep apace of rights granted to minority groups (see *Regents of the University of California* v. *Bakke* 1978; *Kaiser Aluminum and Chemical Corp.* v. *Weber* 1979). The Equal Credit Opportunity Act of 1976 prohibits discrimination in credit transactions on several grounds, including age, but it expressly allows age to be used in computing creditworthiness.

All three laws specifically permit the use of old age as a criterion. It is the beauty of laws outlawing racial discrimination, on the other hand, that they generally forbid consideration of race in a manner that disadvantages racial minorities. If a valid concern affecting racial minorities remains, it must be dealt with by testing for some characteristic less vulnerable than minority status. There is wisdom in denying the use of vulnerable criteria, given the history of discrimination against minority groups; but it is a wisdom forgotten as it applies to the elderly. While the laws tend to prevent the inefficient use of age classification, they do nothing about the efficient but insensitive use of age as a criterion. Undoubtedly many people at age seventy are less useful to their employers than they were at age thirty-five, and we may therefore assume that rational employment policy would have most of them resign to make place for younger workers. Sorting those who should appropriately stay in the job market from those who should retire could be accomplished functionally by predicting probable future performance for all employees, or categorically by having all retire at the age of seventy. One might guess that it was more efficient to do the latter. Yet if race rather than age were the criterion, the former would be compelled. Compulsory retirement and other forms of age discrimination establish every bit as much a badge of inferiority as do racial classifications. In a youth-oriented society, being old leads to being outcast.

The Supreme Court has thought otherwise, at least from a constitutional perspective. Upholding compulsory retirement for fifty-year-old uniformed police officers, the court rejected an equal protection argument made specifically on behalf of police officers but generically of behalf of the elderly. It said:

While the treatment of the aged in this nation has not been wholly free of discrimination, such persons, unlike, say, those who have been discriminated against on the basis of race or national origin, have not experienced a "history of purposeful unequal treatment" or been subjected to unique disabilities on the basis of stereotyped characteristics not truly indicative of their abilities. Old age does not define a "discrete and insular" group, in need of "extraordinary protection from the majoritarian political process." Instead, it marks a stage that each of us will reach if we live out our normal span. Even if the statute could be said to impose a penalty upon a class defined as the aged, it would not impose a distinction sufficiently akin to those classifications that we have found suspect to call for strict judicial scrutiny. (*Massachusetts Board of Retirement* v. *Murgia,* 427 U.S. 307, 313: 1976).

I would urge both the legislative and judicial reexamination of the impact of discrimination on the elderly. My hope is that a more careful review of the problem would lead to more generous treatment of their problems.

Although these are the most important features of law relating directly to aging, legislation has a far greater impact on the elderly in a way which is not expressly age related. The problems I am going to discuss appear applicable to all, but for a variety of reasons single out the elderly as principal victims. As I have already suggested, the aged suffer from a great deprivation of personal autonomy. Even though American society has traditionally protected individual autonomy, until the last decade a second current of state paternalism also ran through social thought and action. The proponents of that paternalism were not concerned with its potential to be more coercive than liberating, but in recent years, the paternalistic model has come increasingly under attack—for just these reasons (Gaylin et al. 1978; Mandell 1975). Challengers emphasize that the preconditions necessary for participation in many public programs are both invasive of individual autonomy and functionally unsound. While society has traditionally focused its attention, in a self-congratulating manner, on the value of providing care for the subject's benefit, little analysis has been devoted to the ultimate "benefit" or to the ramifications of diminished self-determination. Evidence is accumulating that such loss is not negligible, particularly with regard to medical

care. The loss of autonomy may entirely vitiate putative benefits by aggravating the subject's morbidity, and may even
culminate in death.

Several assumptions underlie paternalistic intervention:
first, that it is possible validly to judge that the subject is incompetent to manage personal needs; second, that someone
other than the subject can better determine the content of
those needs; third, that intervention will result in better care
for the subject than would have occurred without intervention;
and finally, that the care provided will be effective, resulting
in an improvement in the subject's quality of life. This chapter
examines the problematical nature of these assumptions as
they function in the areas of personal care and property
management.

General medical treatment is normally provided on a voluntary basis. Save for exceptional situations such as individual
emergency or public danger from contagious disease, competent persons cannot be subjected to the intrusion of medical
procedures without their informed consent (Prosser 1971). A
person possessed of private resources is also free to choose any
form of legally sanctioned medical therapy. It would be un-
thinkable for the majority to impose a particular form of therapy on an independent adult citizen, yet an elderly person who
must obtain needed health care through a medical benefit program or an insurance plan must sacrifice autonomy to conform
to a predetermined therapeutic orientation.

The first assumption underlying such a derogation of autonomy is premised on the recipient's financial impoverishment
and technical ignorance. Older persons are presumed to lack
the necessary knowledge, rather than the necessary rationali-
ty, to determine their own health needs. Licensed professionals, on the other hand, are presumed to possess the requisite
expertise and objectivity to judge effectively and efficiently the
content of the recipient's health needs.

The accuracy of these assumptions is belied by the realities
of the present system. Diagnostic techniques are not as accurate as is commonly supposed (Britton 1974; Sheehan 1978),
rendering the validity of therapeutic programs questionable.
Furthermore, the traditional biochemical model conceives of
disease in physiochemical terms and does not consider the sig-

nificant impact of such psychosocial factors as stress and disruptive personal losses in the development of physical disorders (Bakan 1968; Engel 1977; Holmes and Rahe 1967; Pelletier 1977; Schmale 1958). Yet the elderly are more prone to be afflicted with chronic rather than acute disease (House Select Committee on Aging 1978), and psychosocial factors are particularly implicated in the former. The traditional medical model, therefore, is ill equipped to provide expertise in the evaluation of the older population's health needs. It focuses on acute rather than chronic disease and on curative intervention rather than preventive or supportive measures (House Select Committee on Aging 1976).

Physicians receive little training in stress detection and alleviation or in the relationship of nutrition to disease, although these areas are extremely important to understanding disorders in the elderly. Furthermore, few medical schools provide even a conventionally oriented education in geriatric medicine. Despite these facts, however, both medical benefits programs and health care professionals adhere to the biochemical model. As a result, elderly persons in need of health care are victims of a therapeutic orientation that may be inappropriate to their situation.

Moreover, surrogated decisionmakers cannot be presumed to assess objectively the health needs of the elderly. Medicine has long served to provide "scientific" legitimizations for the social prejudices of the more powerful sector, and this propensity is especially dangerous with respect to the aged. For example, one authority states:

A wide range of myths, stereotypes, and misinformation have interfered with the approach of the health care system to the geriatric patient. Symptoms that elicit concern in younger people are frequently ignored in older ones. As a result, many treatable probems in later life are neither identified nor acknowledged. Instead, they are dismissed as inevitable, irreversible concomitants of the aging process (Cohen 1977, p. 855; see also Butler 1975a, 1975b).

Pathological changes in sleep patterns, for instance, would be explored in a younger person as symptoms of an underlying physical or psychological problem. However, physicians are less likely to pursue the source of such changes in an elderly person, assuming, perhaps, that the elderly normally sleep less. Similarly a nutritional iron deficiency may never be discovered because frailty and confusion are expected in an octogenarian. And insidious congestive heart failure may be termed "fatigue" in a nursing home patient.

The final assumptions supporting covert restrictions of choice—that better care will ensue and that such care will be effective—are the most egregiously defective, particularly as they pertain to the aged. The current structure of medical benefit programs severely limits the freedom of elderly persons to choose care appropriate to their needs and, by strict adherence to the biochemical model, the opportunity for autonomy in hospital and convalescent environments is reduced. The conditions of health benefit and insurance systems, as well as the tax provisions delimiting deductible medical expenses, evince a bias toward institutionalization and technological intervention.

The hospital provides an efficient setting for the cooperation and interaction of specialists, the oversight of their high-technology armamentariums, and the training of fledgling medical students. However, it fosters among elderly patients an attitude of dependency, helplessness, and nonparticipation. Similarly, internment in a nursing home may aggravate a depression syndrome and the sterile atmosphere and lack of stimulation may speed brain deterioration. It is incontrovertible that the disruption caused by institutionalization or relocation is attended by sharp increases in morbidity and mortality among aging persons (Aldrich and Mendkoff 1963; Lieberman 1961; Regan 1972).

Moreover, hospitalization offers a socially sanctioned opportunity to remove an elderly person from home and to insulate those who remain from their personal responsibilities toward that individual, since "better" care is being provided. But better care is not a mere quantum of services; rather, it includes such ineffable factors as love and personal attention. Furthermore, hospitalization may hinder rather than facilitate a salutary outcome by increasing the likelihood of acquiring a disease, often resulting from drug therapy or diagnostic procedures (McLamb and Huntley 1967; Schimmel 1964; Spain

1963). Yet initial hospitalization is frequently a prerequisite for compensation.

Compensation schemes also favor internment in nursing homes and similar facilities, although recent exposés have demonstrated that "good" care in such facilities is the exception rather than the rule. In 1974 the Senate Subcommittee on Long-Term Care deplored the unsanitary, dangerous, and degrading conditions in nursing homes, citing reports of excessive and inappropriate administration of medication, reliance on untrained and unlicensed personnel for direct patient care, and a startling frequency of fires (Senate Special Committee on Aging 1974).

The unfortunate consequences of the conditional benefit programs cannot be characterized as the provision of better care. Such programs have resulted in the inappropriate institutionalization of countless elderly persons, an attrition of available home care services (Ricker-Smith and Trager 1978), and thereby the further foreclosure of alternative care possibilities.

Elderly persons do not have adequate resources to satisfy their health care needs, being particularly victimized by the rising cost of care and the impact of inflation. Therefore, the voluntariness of their participation in conditional benefit programs is quite factitious. General medical treatment is usually not imposed upon competent patients; however, a competency "catch 22" coheres to the rule. That is, an elderly person who refuses the medical treatment proferred through conditional benefit programs risks the use of this refusal as evidence of incompetency and the need for a guardian who would then have the authority to subject the person to the treatment plan. Spouses and children would be especially tempted to initiate such a process in order that the elderly person's health expenditures be covered by the benefit program. An unduly restrictive program, therefore, coerces acceptance of its conditions by bringing together the threat of incompetency proceedings and the pressing need for care.

A modification of perspective is desperately needed. In the future, health benefit programs should seek the widest dissemination of health-oriented information so that freedom of choice may be meaningful: in other words, they should promote the autonomy of the elderly person. Fostering personal participation in the restoration and maintenance of health and motivating mutual cooperation and support within community and family groups will, in all likelihood, serve the best interests of both provider and recipient of the public benefit. Furthermore, evidence is mounting that unconventional or less intrusive care alternatives and therapies are less complicated, less costly, and more beneficial.

Perhaps an alternative scheme, such as a voucher system (see Friedman 1962) that would dispense funds directly to the beneficiary and that would permit a broader range of choice in health services, could ameliorate the present problems. One advantage of the voucher system is that perception of personal autonomy and self-responsibility might have a therapeutic effect. Instructors in biofeedback and meditation techniques, for instance, report that when patients discover their ability to control autonomic physical functions, they are often motivated to improve other aspects of their lives, such as dietary habits (Pelletier 1977). Similarly, a study in which a group of elderly nursing home residents were encouraged to be self-responsible reported an increase in activity, sociability, and general satisfaction among the tested group as compared with the control group, to whom the responsibility of the nursing staff for patient welfare had been emphasized (Langer and Rodin 1976).

The most flagrant examples of overt intervention into the life of an older person result from guardianship and involuntary civil commitment procedures. Such intrusions are commonly premised on the best interests of the subjects and directly wrest personal control from elderly persons, ostensibly to improve the quality of their lives. The process of psychiatric intervention begins with a decision that the elderly individual, because of a mental disorder, is either unable to provide adequately for basic needs or is otherwise in need of treatment. The decision to intervene may be simple and nonadjudicative or it may involve an elaborate judicial hearing. Each state and the federal government have their own forms of guardianship and civil commitment (see American Bar Association Committee on the Mentally Disabled 1979; Mental Disability Resource Center 1979). Some states have more than one type of guardianship; for example, California has both conservatorship and guardianship. The procedures and consequences of guardianship differ as well as the names. In many states they include the possibility of long-term institutionalization. In California, on the other hand, no psychiatric hospitalization is permitted unless a proceeding is separately brought for that purpose. Once intervention is authorized, under either guardianship or civil commitment procedures, elderly persons may be treated, within varying limits, irrespective of their articulated wishes (Plotkin 1978).

The determination that older persons are unable to care for themselves is essentially a predicative judgment drawn from an assessment of an individual's present condition and past behavior. This judgment avers that the person will, as a result of "mental disease," be unable to choose to provide for his or her own personal needs. The judgment of mental disease/inability-to-provide is viewed as a medical diagnosis/prognosis effectively within the province of the medical profession, since the model of mental illness is commonly assimilated to the bio-medical model of physical illness (Szasz 1970, 1974; Szasz and Alexander 1972). Great reliance is therefore placed on the testimony of psychiatrists, in all stages of the decisionmaking process.

There is growing evidence, however, that psychiatrists are unable reliably to diagnose the status of mental illness in their patients (Ennis and Litwack 1974). The literature further demonstrates that psychiatrists have neither the training nor the expertise to predict a person's proclivity for violence to others or to self (Dersowitz 1968). By analogy, such evidence of diagnostic confusion regarding dangerousness suggests a likelihood that psychiatrists may be inaccurate in predicting capacity for self-sufficiency as well. This inadequacy of predictive skills is magnified by psychiatrists' evident tendency toward overprediction of both dangerousness and need for treatment. The failure to predict future harm may expose the professional to ridicule, legal action, loss of reputation, and personal guilt should the subject, upon release, injure himself or others. Involuntary intervention, on the other hand, insulates the decisionmaker from future criticism. Moreover, many psychiatrists err on the side of intervention since, in their view, the result is at worst the provision of treatment. In recent years, however, a rising awareness has developed, catalyzed by dramatic litigation, that institutionalization results in severe debilitation and stigmatization as well as a massive loss of liberty.

The second assumption underlying involuntary intervention—that a surrogate decisionmaker can effectively determine the best interests of the elderly person—is also doubtful. Such a surrogate, it is supposed, most likely can help the older person achieve a normative state; that is, the person may be housed, clothed, fed, and cared for "more satisfactorily"—but "satisfaction" is defined by parties other than the individual. This putative improvement in circumstances may carry with it the detrimental effects of the person's perceived loss of liberty and autonomy.

Furthermore, the present system of substitute decisionmaking presents the danger of unrecognized, and therefore unchallenged, adverse interests. Psychiatrists may impose treatment not only to protect their patients, but also to preserve their professional control. Myriad other adverse interests may be disguised beneath an ostensible concern for the subject's welfare. Children, for example, may desire to remove an elderly parent from their home because the situation proves disruptive or bothersome. Moreover, the facade of altruism deflects attention from the reality of interests adverse to the subject, allowing the decisionmakers to function without impediment (see Alexander 1977; Alexander and Lewin 1972). The inherent potential for conflicting interests suggests that caution be exercised in assuming that a surrogate decisionmaker will genuinely pursue the best interests of the elderly subject.

In addition, these intrusive measures cannot be justified by the purported objectivity and competence of surrogate decisionmakers. For example, the aged are presently overrepresented in the population of involuntary mental patients. Regan (1972) has observed that "the percentage of mental-hospital first admissions of elderly persons is increasing more rapidly than the total population of the aged," and that the aged make up 30 percent of mental hospital patients (p. 574).

It is unclear to what extent these statistics simply reflect increased debility in the aged, nor is it known how many such patients have nonpsychiatric medical problems. Unfortunately, like so many psychiatric diagnoses, nonpsychiatric diagnoses also tend to reflect the expectations of those who bring patients to the diagnostician. "Dad is just not himself," "Mom is so much more forgetful," "Dad's leg is giving him so much more trouble"—these and similar statements provide a strong impression for a physician who may not have previously seen the patient and who has had experience with patients who were out of touch with their own functioning.

This situation is exacerbated by the fact that physicians and psychiatrists are inclined to posit an inexorable correlation between senescence and senility. The label of "senility" is misapplied with alarming frequency, although studies indicate that fewer than 5 percent of persons over sixty-five manifest true senile- dementia (Cohen 1977; National Institute of Aging 1978; President's Commission on Mental Health 1978). Brain syndrome is considered acute if reversible, and chronic if otherwise. Acute brain syndrome may, however, mask such physical or mental conditions as simple depression, vitamin deficiency, traumatic injury, or a variety of other ills. If the underlying condition is not treated, deterioration may in fact confirm the original diagnosis of brain syndrome (Busse 1973; Goldfarb 1975). A brain syndrome diagnosis in general, and certainly a chronic brain syndrome diagnosis in particular, may therefore be a self-fulfilling prophecy. A National Institute on Aging Task Force estimates that at least 300,000 persons afflicted with dementia could have been restored to useful life by appropriate evaluation and treatment. Moreover, the diagnosis may mask needed treatment in a less dramatic way. For example, a colleague recently discussed a situation in which his mother had suffered a stroke. She made a miraculous recovery: all but bladder function returned to normal. The treating physician was pleased, so pleased in fact that it did not occur to him to investigate the cause of the remaining problem. At my colleague's insistence, however, the physician continued to search for the cause and eventually found a massive infection that quickly responded to treatment. The patient was cured of all symptoms.

Much of the initial data on which mental health diagnosticians act in these cases concerns behavior. In brain syndrome, a previously healthy individual suddenly becomes disturbed, confused, restless, or disoriented. Because a significant portion of chronic brain syndrome diagnosis is comparative, data must be matched against the patient's prior mental history. Most of the behavioral symptoms on which a decision must be made will already have taken place by the time the physician sees the patient, and therefore heavy reliance must be placed on an informer's observation of the person's conduct. The opportunity for bias on the informer's part is obvious. Just as an incompetency proceeding can be used to indicate the petitioner's interest in the finances of an older person, so too can information about older persons' behaviors be used to cast them as sufficiently debilitated to require involuntary treatment.

Informants may not necessarily be conscious of their role, nor may they necessarily be lying. The entire inquiry is so unclear that it is possible to paint a picture of gross disability simply by selective recollections, however innocent, of recent events. The diagnosis in turn reflects the same vague standards. One researcher reports that 77.7 percent of first-time geriatric admissions during one year's time were admitted for brain syndrome (Wang 1969). Another study of diagnoses of patients over sixty-five on first admissions to mental hospitals in Toronto, New York, and London found the respective percentages to be 41.8 percent in Canada, 79.8 percent in New York, and 42.8 percent in England. The study concluded that the difference in percentages was probably not the result of differences in patients, but rather differences in the diagnostic bias of U.S. physicians (Duckworth and Ross 1975). In Canada and England, the percentages of functional (nonorganic) disorders were comparably higher. Because there is a wide textbook difference between nonorganic dysfunction and organic brain syndrome, these discrepancies indicate some reason for skepticism about chronic brain syndrome diagnoses.

The assumptions underlying involuntary intervention are not separable by bright, conceptual lines. Particularly inextricable are several assumptions already noted: that better care will ensue by virtue of the intervention, and that such care will result in a higher quality of life for the subject. In recent years, the deplorable conditions in state mental institutions and nursing homes have been exposed and decried. The past decade has seen a silent exodus of patients from these institutions, and many remaining facilities have improved their physical conditions. The system nonetheless remains profoundly inadequate. Discharged patients often live in circumstances as lamentable as those formerly existing in the large institutions (Senate Special Committee on Aging 1974), and the persons who remain in institutions continue to suffer from a paucity of appropriate care and individual attention. The effects of this chronic inadequacy of resources are exacerbated by the degrading impact of the institutional routine and the depersonalizing attitudes of service providers toward patients.

Numerous studies attest to the danger of involuntary intervention for the aging (Blenkner 1967). A Benjamin Rose Institute report (1974), for instance, has suggested that intrusion beyond basic housekeeping assistance may produce more detriment than benefit. While concluding that the most traumatic form of protective service was involuntary placement, the report attempted to discern the efficacy of all protective services, not just involuntary placement. The study went on to note, however, that service increases the likelihood of institutionalization: "Experienced social workers appear to have a strong tendency to move old people into 'protective settings' when assigned responsibility for their welfare" (p. 138). According to the initial study: "One must conclude on the basis of data gathered from following up ... service and control cases the project service was not effective in slowing down deterioration and physical functioning—two major reasons frequently given for intervening in a protective case" (pp. 68–69). The study's alarming conclusion was that protective services did not lengthen life; on the contrary, they appeared to shorten people's lives. The hypothesis was later restudied and reconfirmed. At the conclusion of the second study, it was noted:

Taking the findings as a whole it is difficult to avoid the conclusion that (a) participants in the experimental service program were institutionalized earlier than they would have otherwise been and (b) that this earlier institutionalization did not—contrary to intent—prove protective in terms of survival of the older person although it did relieve collaterals and community agents (p. 157).

The most egregious aspects of this system of involuntary intervention on personal care could be mitigated by several practicable changes. First, the limited competence that is available to society through both lawyers and physicians should be applied in a reordered fashion to maximize its benefit. Lawyers should be absolutely prohibited (in fact, a proper interpretation of ethical considerations already prohibits them) from undertaking to represent a person, and then later petitioning for anyone's involuntary intervention in the client's affairs. If there are people to deal with involuntary intervention, they should be people trained in social work, psychology, psychiatry, or some similar field. Since psychiatrists have difficulty knowing when to resort to involuntary process, lawyers should certainly not attempt the task.

Correlatively, the law should limit psychiatrists and psychologists to dealing with the issue they can address best: treatability. There is no reason why anyone not treatable should ever be hospitalized, and there is no reason why a physician ought ever to be involved in deciding whether a person can function in property management, or determine danger to society, or related fields, since those issues are similar to other questions of fact with which lawyers customarily deal.

However, the most difficult question, given our present concern for responsibility, cannot be resolved by simply assigning to the two principal professors the areas they handle best. What is to be done with the "irresponsible persons" who may resist treatment or surrogate property management as part of the mental condition for which we would hold them irresponsible? The question does not allow an easy answer that is socially acceptable. My answer would be that the best available way of dealing with the problem is to accept what a person says, whether the person is considered competent or incompetent in other respects. Since the solution may be out of line with current notions, a modest proposal may be more acceptable: every person would still be the ultimate judge of whether intervention is to take place in his or her life. The test would become: "What would the person have done if competent to decide?"

The idea is not a new one. Several states have recently adopted laws allowing people to direct that their lives not be artificially maintained when survival becomes impossible and when they can no longer be consulted. It is only a short step from such a declaration to a further declaration respecting what to do if, in the future, a person were found to be incompetent to make decisions (see Alexander 1979). Some will no doubt choose to authorize intervention. In fact, such authorization statements are already in limited use. Others will certainly choose to reject such intervention. To keep legal issues to a minimum, a statement as to future desire should probably become incontestable after a year or two. Otherwise one would always have to go back to the question of whether the person were competent to make the original statement. It is probable that society can live with a system in which people who have not been in a psychiatric hospital for, say, a year or so can have their written wishes honored as to whether now to hospitalize. Similarly, wishes with respect to surrogate management of property can be honored.

Of course, most persons will not execute a statement either for or against involuntary intervention. Even for them, however, the question of what they would have requested had they made a statement is the best available issue on which to determine intervention. The issue of what a person would have done is clearly a legal, not a medical, issue. Lawyers can presumably focus on conduct evidencing a desire for help or rejecting medical treatment in other contexts. As far as hospitalization is concerned, physicians would then have the opportunity to determine whether they can be of benefit should the person be hospitalized. Both groups would do what they do best.

The assumption that it is possible validly to judge the competence of an elderly person is as problematical in regard to property management as to personal care. Again the judgment of incompetency necessarily involves an attempt to predict future conduct: the judicial process tends to accord great deference to the testimony of experts, and a scientific basis for prediction has not been demonstrated to exist.

Furthermore, the ambiguous standards of the substantive law in guardianship proceedings—a problem that similarly inheres in all adjudications concerning involuntary intervention for personal care—preclude effective application of procedural due process analysis. The standard pertaining to the appropriate ability to manage property is unclear and allows a broad scope of discretion to the court or jury. The due process model cannot overcome such frailty of the substantive: the model can be effective only in preventing injustice in situations where the operative standards are narrowly drawn. At present, when vague conditions of incompetency prevail, and medical testimony is effectively determinative, procedural due process obfuscates the deficiency of this assumption by lending a deceptive gloss of validity to the proceeding.

As previously discussed, the justifications for paternalistic intervention in the life of an older person are premised in part on the apparent objectivity and benevolence of the surrogate decisionmaker. Once again, however, such altruistic disinterestedness cannot be lightly presumed. Those who are potential beneficiaries of the elderly individual's affluence take a natural interest in its waste; in turn, the state has an interest in preventing its citizens from so reducing their financial integrity as to become public charges. Even though these interests are adverse to those of the ward, the present process, with its focus on benefit to the ward, inadequately and inarticulately deals with such adverse interests. In consequence, beneficiaries find themselves in the cynical position of being forced to plead in court for surrogate management premised on benefit to the object of the proceeding rather than, candidly, benefit to themselves. Unfortunately, when the underlying self-interest of the petitioners is probed they often appear in a very bad light in such court proceedings. Equally unfortunately, when this issue is not explored, potential beneficiaries may be awarded an interest in the ward's property that the court would find untenable from the perspective of protecting the beneficiaries' interest rather than the ward's.

Of course, avarice is not the only factor adverse to the interests of the ward; persons may also seek to have guardianship declared for administrative convenience. For this reason, apparently, the states of California and New York are active petitioners for guardianship of large numbers of people (see Alexander and Lewin 1972). Having the power to sign documents on behalf of their wards is obviously quite useful. A similar kind of utility may well attend to familial relations in the absence of an extensive estate. Clearly, many interests play a significant role in the decisionmaking process.

It is important to recognize that, however benevolent the intention of those who would seek to substitute other decisionmakers for the aged, persons deprived of the right to decide for themselves will have lost the fairly basic attribute of citizenship. Consequently, it seems more appropriate to view the question of how the law should intervene, not as a question of maximizing benefit to the potential ward, but of reducing to a minimum the deprivation of that person's rights. From this perspective, one might better ask in whose interest is a surrogate manager of property appointed?

There is one sense in which it seems reasonable to view the surrogate as chosen solely in the ward's own interests. Since there are usually people of greater skill and capacity than any given person, courts could probably find property managers for most people who, because of superior experience and skill, would better manage the property than their wards. Without even considering whether the legal process is perfect enough to substitute a better decisionmaker in most cases—a dubious proposition—it is easy to reject the notion of benefit to a person occasioned by providing such paternalistic oversight. We may, of course, always voluntarily obtain a skilled manager for our property; if one is involuntarily imposed, however, we should be skeptical of the benefit of such appointment to the potential ward.

Especially in the case of the aged, one can reject the facile answer that a surrogate can preserve property that the ward will later be able to use. To the extent that conditions of the aged are likely to result from general mental deterioration, it seems unlikely that property management would often revert to the ward. Although a ward's wealth may increase, unless the individual retains the power to spend money for his or her own enjoyment, the ward hardly seems likely to perceive affluence as a benefit. It is, of course, theoretically possible that a condition requiring substitute management is temporary, and that the ward may benefit from an intervention that safeguards property which could later be enjoyed, but experience indicates that this rarely occurs.

The coupling of management operations and decisionmaking in the hands of the surrogate manager may, in any event, interfere unnecessarily with the rights of the ward. As many of the aged suffer merely from memory loss and unfamiliarity with legal processes without having lost their judgment concerning their personal goals, a provision allowing a surrogate to seize decisionmaking authority appears to be an overreaction to the problem. As an alternative to guardians or conservators, the law should permit courts to appoint a new category of agents called, perhaps, "legal assistants."

Legal assistants would be responsible for reviewing with their charges all major financial transactions. They would remind the ward of prior obligations, legal restrictions, and other complications to be anticipated but would be expressly denied the right to substitute their own decisions for that of their charges. In effect, they would provide a service that is directly responsive to a weak memory and a lack of orientation to the legal framework of commerce without removing the essential right to property disposition from the aged person.

Social tensions and conceptual conflicts have begun to cause the disintegration and dismantlement of the present system, a process reflected in the trend of new legislation that has rapidly moved from allowing open-ended intervention to requiring that intervention last only for fixed periods of time. The best illustration comes from California's Lanterman-Petris-Short Act (1972), which is not a guardianship law at all, but relates to involuntary hospitalization. In it, all involuntary commitments are made for very short periods of time, except for persons theoretically totally unable to function, the so-called gravely disabled. Procedures are provided for extending those periods of time through court proceedings, but these extending procedures are very rarely used. Furthermore, initial empirical study suggests that short-term intervention is no less effective than the prior indefinite intervention. If future studies confirm the initial results, it will probably become much more difficult to justify long-term intervention.

During 1977 probate conservatorships were altered in California by the Lanterman Bill, incorporating much of the philosophy of the Lanterman-Petris-Short Act into the probate code. A previous study by the National Senior Citizens Center had determined that 80 percent of persons for whom conservatorship had been ordered were over sixty-five. In addition, the study found that 93 percent of these people had been conserved without their appearance in court. Finally, the study noted that 97 percent had been conserved without legal representation in the proceedings. The new bill was designed to assure that the elderly would no longer be the objects of such casual deprivations of their liberty.

As the Lanterman-Petris-Short Act had done before it, the new Lanterman Bill established strong procedural safeguards against improperly obtained conservatorships. Chief among these safeguards was a provision that prohibited, in most circumstances, granting orders of conservatorship or guardianship in the absence of the ward. Another provision required a court investigator to visit the proposed ward in those infrequent circumstances where the ward has been certified as unable to attend the hearing. Review provisions for conservatorships and guardianships were more stringent than those under prior law, and notice and hearing provisions were strengthened. Finally, under the new bill, the vague standards that allowed the appointment of guardians and conservators because of the infirmities of old age have been abolished. The new law makes clear that the standard is functional and nonmedical, allowing appointment of a surrogate when a person is considered "substantially unable to manage his own financial resources or resist fraud or undue influence." The law limits the application of the new standard by providing that isolated instances of fraud or undue influence should not suffice as proof of incapacity.

Clearly, the present system of surrogate decisionmaking is undergoing a transformation, but several salutary proposals have yet to be implemented.

First, the law should be rewritten to eliminate vindication of adverse interests. If, for example, there are persons with a legitimate concern about inheriting from an older person who is presently squandering money, the law should either recognize that interest (as it does the interest of a creditor in debt payment, a wife in postmarital support, the state in having its tax bills paid) or should make it clear that it does not recognize them. In any event, all people having an interest should be allowed to protect their interest to the same extent that, for example, creditors presently protect their interest through legal proceedings. No one would be required to go to court to talk about the best interests of their debtor.

Correspondingly, the law should be written to remove all financial incentives for bringing guardianship proceedings. It is impracticable to attempt to determine the role of avarice on a case-by-case basis. Equally, administrative sloth has made states large-scale petitioners. Perhaps legal disincentives could be created, making guardianship responsibilities even more burdensome to administrators and making devolution of property even more difficult for beneficiaries than under present intestate succession.

Another solution to the problem could be to require courts to obtain professional managers as surrogates in all cases. In the event the estate is sizable, the task should not be difficult. (In the event that the estate is too small to attract professional management, the temptation to near relatives is likely also less pronounced.) If professional management is available, a court should give near relatives the option of professional management or their own appointment, on condition that they expressly renounce any financial benefit from the ward, in his life or on his death, other than the fee for guardianship or conservatorship. If professional management is unavailable, no such renunciation should be required. Of course, the previously expressed wishes of the ward, if legally competent, ought to prevail over the plan described. The plan is designed to meet what will likely remain the great majority of cases in which wards have not previously expressed themselves on the subject.

It is rather curious that in a legal system that ordinarily is very cognizant of checks and balances, persons are allowed the weapon of incompetency in promoting self-interest. Even elemental notions about conflicts of interests suggest that a revision of the underlying theory is long overdue. Where intervention is required for any reason, it seems extremely important to assure that if surrogates are to be appointed they be as free of avarice as the system will allow. It should be clear that a surrogate's obligation is to maximize the benefit to the ward and not to the ward's heirs. At the same time, the system should be recast to reduce the occasions for the appointment of a surrogate at all.

In many ways, the elderly are victims of intended benevolence. The problems of aging have been misunderstood, and the "remedies" have rarely been critically evaluated. Many of these issues relate to the general society as well, but the programs hurt the elderly especially because of their physical and economic vulnerability. In contrast, by expanding options and reducing involuntary intervention for the elderly, everyone will benefit.

REFERENCES

Aldrich and Mendkoff. 1963. "Relocation of the Aged and Disabled: A Mortality Study." *Journal of the American Geriatrics Society* 11:185.

Alexander, G.J. 1977. "On Being Imposed upon by Artful or Designing Persons: The California Experience with the Involuntary Placement of the Aged." *San Diego Law Review* 14:1083.

Alexander, G.J. 1979. "Premature Probate: A Different Perspective on Guardianship for the Elderly." *Stanford Law Review* 31:1003.

Alexander, G.J., and T. Lewin. 1972. *The Aged and the Need for Surrogate Management.* Syracuse: Syracuse University Press.

American Bar Association Committee on the Mentally Disabled. 1979. Developmental Disabilities State Legislative Project. *Guardianship and Conservatorship.* Washington, D.C.: A.B.A. Committee on the Mentally Disabled.

Bakan, D. 1968. *Disease, Pain and Sacrifice.* Boston: Beacon Press.

Benjamin Rose Institute. 1967. *Progress Report on Protective Services for Older People.* Cleveland: Benjamin Rose Institute.

Benjamin Rose Institute. 1974. *Protective Services for Older People: Findings from the Benjamin Rose Institute Study.* Cleveland: Benjamin Rose Institute.

Blenkner, M. 1967. "Environmental Change and the Aging Individual." *Gerontologist* 7:101.

Britton, M. 1974. "Diagnostic Errors Discovered at Autopsy." *Acta Medica Scandanavica* 196:203.

Busse, E. 1973. "Mental Disorder in Later Life: Organic Brain Syndrome." In *Mental Illness in Later Life,* edited by E. Busse and E. Pfeiffer. Washington, D.C.: American Psychiatric Association.

Butler, R.N. 1975a. "Psychiatry and the Elderly: An Overview." *American Journal of Psychology* 132:893.

Butler, R. 1975b. *Why Survive? Being Old in America.* New York: Harper & Row.

Cohen, G.D. 1977. "Approach to the Geriatric Patient." *Medical Clinics of North America* 61:855.

Dersowitz, A.M. 1968. "Psychiatry in the Legal Process: A Knife that Cuts Both Ways." *Trial* 4:29.

Duckworth, G.S., and H. Ross. 1975. "Diagnostic Differences in Psychogeriatric Patients in Toronto, New York and London, England." *Canadian Medical Association Journal* 112:847.

Engel, G.L. 1977. "The Need for a New Medical Model: A Challenge for Biomedicine." *Science* 196:129.

Ennis, B.J., and T.R. Litwack. 1974. "Psychiatry and the Presumption of Expertise: Flipping Coins in the Courtroom." *California Law Review* 62:693.

Friedman, M. 1962. *Capitalism and Freedom.* Chicago: University of Chicago Press.

Gaylin, W.; I. Glasser; S. Marcus; and D. Rothman. 1978. *Doing Good.* New York: Pantheon Press.

Goldfarb, A.I. 1975. "Memory and Aging." In *The Physiology and Pathology of Human Aging,* edited by R. Goldman and M. Rockstein, p. 149. New York: Academic Press.

Holmes, T.H., and R.H. Rahe. 1967. "The Social Readjustment Rating Scale." *Journal of Psychosomatic Research* 11:213.

House Select Committee on Aging. 1976. *New Perspectives in Health Care for Older Americans.* Washington, D.C.: Government Printing Office.

House Select Committee on Aging. 1978. *Future of Health Care and the Elderly.* Washington, D.C.: Government Printing Office.

Langer, E.J., and J. Rodin. 1976. "The Effects of Choice and Enhanced Personal Responsibility for the Aged: A Field Experiment in an Institutional Setting." *Journal of Personality and Social Psychology* 34:191.

———. *Mental Disability Law Reporter* 1979, vol. 3. Washington, D.C.: A.B.A. Mental Disability Resource Center.

Lieberman, M.A. 1961. "Relationship of Mortality Rates to Entrance for a Home for the Aged." *Geriatrics* 16:515.

McLamb, and Huntley. 1967. "The Hazards of Hospitalization." *Southern Medical Journal* 60:100.

Mandell, B., ed. 1975. *Welfare in America.* Englewood Cliffs, New Jersey: Prentice-Hall.

National Institute of Aging, National Institutes of Health. 1978. *Treatable Dementia in the Elderly.* Bethesda, Maryland: National Institutes of Health.

Pelletier, K. 1977. *Mind as Healer, Mind as Slayer.* New York: Dell.

Plotkin, R. 1978. "Limiting the Therapeutic Orgy: Mental Patients' Right to Refuse Treatment." *Northwestern University Law Review* 72:461.

President's Commission on Mental Health. 1978. *Report of the Task Panel on the Mental Health of the Elderly.* Washington, D.C.: Government Printing Office.

Prosser, W. 1971. *Law of Torts,* 4th edition. St. Paul, Minnesota: West.

Regan, J.J. 1972. "Protective Services for the Elderly: Commitment, Guardianship, and Alternatives." *William and Mary Law Review* 13:569, 588–89.

Ricker-Smith, K., and B. Trager. 1978. "In-Home Health Services in California." *Medical Care* 16:173.

Schimmel, E.U. 1964. "The Hazards of Hospitalization." *Annuals of Internal Medicine* 60:100.

Schmale, A.H. 1958. "Relationship of Separation and Depression to Disease." *Psychosomatic Medicine* 20:259.

Senate Special Committee on Aging. 1974. *Nursing Home Care in the United States: Failure in Public Policy, Introductory Report.* Washington, D.C.: Government Printing Office.

Sheehan, M.W. 1978. "Diagnostic Errors in Clinical Practice." *Texas Medicine* 74:92.

Spain, D. 1963. *The Complications of Modern Medical Practice.* New York: Grune & Stratton.

Szasz, T. 1970. *Ideology and Insanity.* New York: Doubleday.

Szasz, T. 1974. *The Myths of Mental Illness,* 2nd edition. New York: Harper & Row.

Szasz, T., and G.J. Alexander. 1972. "Law, Property and Psychiatry." *American Journal of Ortho-Psychology* 42:610.

U.S. Department of Health, Education and Welfare. 1977. *Health: United States 1976-1977.* Washington, D.C.: Government Printing Office.

Wang. 1969. "Organic Brain Syndromes." In *Behavior and Adaptation in Later Life,* edited by E. Busse and E. Pfeiffer, pp. 263, 265. Washington, D.C.: American Psychiatric Association.

4 OLD WIVES' TALES

Anne Firor Scott

Is there anything left to be said about aging? Everywhere one looks it seems to be topic A—or at least running a close second to death and dying—for the attention of newspapers, columnists, television, publishers, the government, and the universities. At least three college alumni magazines have devoted attention to the subject recently—winding up, of course, with lots of handy advice on estate planning! If one boils down all the statistics, digests all the viewings-with-alarm, the exhortations to be up and jogging, and all the rest, three basic and intractable facts emerge which set the stage for my own examination of the topic.

First, whether we like it or not, our population is getting older. When George Washington was inaugurated, half the people in this country were under sixteen, and only a tiny handful were over sixty-five. Being president must have been something like being head of Boys' Town. Now thirty is the halfway point, and 10 percent of the population is past age sixty-five—and being president is not so much fun anymore. Furthermore, this trend is bound to continue, and unless someone slips up with a nuclear weapon, or lets loose some anthrax germs, or dumps one more lethal chemical in the Mississippi, the population will continue to grow older. This, we might say, is society's problem.

Second, looking at the same set of facts from the perspective of the individual, more and more of us will live a long time. Of every hundred persons born the year Washington took office, only twenty reached the age of seventy. Of every hundred children born this year (again, failing some manmade disaster), eighty will live past their seventieth birthdays. There are more Americans over age sixty-five alive at this moment than the total of all the people who reached that age in all the years that have gone before. So lots of people are going to have to learn to live as elder persons, and this we might define as the individual's problem.

Third, in each age group past forty-five there are more women than men, and by the time one reaches seventy-five, there are 156 women for every 100 men. I'm not certain whose problem that is, but I am pretty sure it is one reason for considering the subject of women in a series on aging.

Aging is not solely a biological process. People live in particular historical circumstances, and the interaction between individuals and the society in which they happen to be born and grow up determines the special characteristics of their experience. Let us begin, then, by examining the broad social changes that have taken place in the way American women have lived and worked since the seventeenth century, asking how those changes have affected the process of aging and the experience of being an old woman. It has been nearly four centuries since the first women arrived in Jamestown, in response to the heartfelt cry of the men who were already there that they had nobody to do their washing. What can we learn from the experience of all the women who have preceded us that bears on the three problems I outlined in the beginning?

Those early Jamestown settlers and their successors for the next 200 years became partners in a domestic economy. That is to say, men, women, and children all worked together to make the family living—and *make* is indeed the correct verb, since the family created with its own hands most of what it consumed. There was always a clear sexual division of labor. Men chopped down trees, plowed and planted, built cabins, harvested crops. Women kept gardens, took care of poultry, milked cows, churned butter, made cheese, spun, wove, and sewed cloth, preserved and prepared the family food, took care of sick people, and, if they were literate themselves, taught the children their ABCs. Artisans' wives learned their husbands' craft in order to carry on if he became ill or died.

Healthy women were pregnant on the average of every two years until menopause, and though many children died in infancy or early childhood, enough survived to bring about very rapid population growth. Some families were large. We hear a great deal about colonial women dying in childbirth, and many did. However, so many men died of smallpox, yellow fever, pneumonia, tuberculosis, and other ailments that even in the eighteenth century there were times and places where widows outnumbered widowers (Keyssar 1974).

Old age was an experience confined to a small proportion of all those born in the eighteenth and nineteenth centuries, but of the 20 percent who lived to age seventy, many lived into their eighties, nineties, and beyond. The *American Register*, a sort of early version of *Time*, regularly carried a list of people in various parts of the country who had passed the one hundred mark, with as much detail as could be gathered about their lives. For these truly aged folks social security lay almost entirely in the family, with the town government and the poorhouse as the last resort.

Colonial men were careful to provide support for surviving wives in their wills. Leaving the family house and land to a son, the father spelled out his widow's entitlements: "the parlor end of the house . . . with the cellar that hath lock and key to it," "free liberty to bake, brew and wash etc. in the kitchen," plenty of wood for her stove "ready cut and at her door," such furniture as she might need: "bedstead . . . bedding . . . the best green rug . . . the best low chair . . . and a good cushion." She might also be provided a cow or chickens and some help in taking care of them: the cow, for example, "to be brought into the yard daily" for her to milk. Sometimes she was to have a fixed share of apples and pears and a gentle horse to ride to church. Sometimes she was to have regular payments in wheat and corn, or books from her husband's library. The one I like best is the provision that she shall have "beer, as she hath now" (Demos 1978). For a long time I worried about the lack of faith in filial responsibility which these wills seem to reflect, until it dawned on me that the suspicion probably rested less on the sons than upon the daughters-in-law (Freeman 1899 contains some insightful short stories that illuminate this subject).

A woman who bore her last child at the age of forty-five did not have to worry much about an empty nest. Indeed, one eighteenth century woman doubtless spoke for many when she wrote in her journal: "I have often thought . . . that women who live to get over the time of Childbareing if other things are favourable to them, experience more comfort and satisfaction than at any other period of their lives" (Drinker 1797).

Such was the mortality of the age, however, that orphaned grandchildren or great-grandchildren were not uncommon. Benjamin Franklin's favorite sister, for example, in her seventies found herself taking care of three very young great-grandchildren whose mother had died in bearing her fourth child in four years. Franklin's sister wrote him that the children probably needed "some person more lively and Patient to watch over them continually," but since no such person volunteered, she did it anyway, and without complaint (Van Doren 1950). When the children were finally off her hands, she retired to a little house in Boston with a favorite granddaughter for a companion and wrote her brother a complete description of her life. She spoke thankfully of having a warm house, a good bed, plenty to eat, neighbors to visit, the companionship of her grandchild, and then she added: "When I look around me on all my acquaintance I do not see won I have reason to think happier than I am and would not change my neighbour with my Self where will you find one in a more comfortable State as I see Every won has their Trobles and I sopose them to be such as fitts them best & shakeing off them might be only changing for the wors."

This was a woman who had borne twelve children and watched eleven of them die, who had been driven from her home during the Revolution, and who had often in her long life had to work very hard to provide food and clothing for her children, grandchildren, and great-grandchildren. The fervor of her appreciation for food, heat, and kind company suggest that such amenities could not be taken for granted by elder persons, especially women, in her day. Indeed some poor widows among her contemporaries were being told to leave certain New England towns and villages because the town fathers did not want them to be a burden on the taxpayers. It is hard to imagine where such women went or how they survived.

If we turn from our very meager information about the realities of women's lives in those early days to the question of how women were defined by the society, we can find a few clues. The law provides one index of social attitudes, and a woman who was married had no independent legal existence. Common law viewed husband and wife as one, and that one the man. Women's property as well as their persons belonged to their husbands. They could neither vote nor serve on juries, nor determine the guardianship of their children.

Another index of status is the availability of education. At the most basic level there were far more illiterate women than illiterate men, and at the highest level, none of the nine colonial colleges admitted women to study. Indeed one colonial governor had told his friends that a certain woman in his town had gone mad from reading books and doing other things he considered unbecoming a female. Ministers and other self-appointed advisors counseled women to defer to their husbands in all things and warned them that a public difference of opinion with a husband was a calamity to be avoided at all cost.

It is no wonder that some lively and strong-minded women chose to remain single. For example, Susanna Wright, a Quaker woman living in western Pennsylvania, was well known as a kind of home-grown lawyer, medical advisor, and general counselor to the community. She was also a champion of the rights of Indians. Considering that she was born in 1697, I was rather intrigued to find that though one Samuel Blunston had repeatedly asked her to marry him, she preferred simply to live as his closest friend and to manage his affairs. Evidently "meaningful relationships" were not invented in the twentieth century. Upon his death he left her all his possessions (Biddle and Lowrie 1942).

When we come to ask specifically how aged women were viewed, we have less information. From what one can surmise, a great deal depended on social class. A woman who had property to dispose of could count on more respect than a poor widow who might become dependent on the town or her children for support. Not all widows were as realistic as one in South Carolina who noted in a letter to her son: "The death of... Parents who leave property is considered more a gain than a loss" (Mathis 1979).

Respect also appears to have been a function of usefulness. A grandmother able to spin, weave, churn, and mind the children was more likely to be a valued member of the family than one who sat in the chimney corner complaining about the cold and the younger generation (James and James 1971).

If we turn to linguistic evidence, I regret to say that I have found no female equivalent for the word "sage," but there are an unsettling number of times when one finds old women being called hag, crone, or witch. And indeed in Salem, old women were actually accused of being witches and hanged. One must conclude that poor women, especially those who were servants or slaves, had a very hard time of it if they outlived their capacity for useful work.

In summary, woman's life in what we nowadays call the preindustrial society was not an easy one. Whether she was an ordinary farmer's wife working from daylight to dark, or married to a wealthy planter with responsibility for the clothing and feeding and medical care of many slaves, whether she was the wife of a small craftsman who helped in the shop and learned his trade, or whether she was one of those who set out for the backwoods and helped her husband clear a field and build a cabin, she had little time to worry about her condition. Without women's labor the economy could not have been built as rapidly as it was, and certainly America would not have been so rapidly populated that by 1776 it was ready to cast off from the main ship and become independent. As for aging women, two in ten made it to age seventy, and for those two the quality of life depended on the economic situation of the whole family connection, on the personalities of their children, and on the woman's own energy and disposition.

From this glimpse of what we do and do not know about our preindustrial forbears, let us take a large leap into the late nineteenth century when the country was in the throes of transformation from a rural to an urban-industrial society. Let us ask: What did that great change mean for women? Until 1920 half our population continued to live on farms, and for farm wives the situation was much as it had been earlier, for they continued to perform essential manual labor and to thrive or wilt depending on the family's total economic situation and their own health and disposition.

For the growing number of women who lived in towns and cities, however, the structure of daily life was changing in fundamental ways. It is important to note that the majority of urban dwellers were wage earners, who often lived on the margin of subsistence. Many were immigrants. It was usually necessary for married women in this segment of the population to contribute to the family income, either by working for wages outside their homes or by taking in what was called "home work"—stitching shoes or clothing or making hats in their own houses. Failing all else, wives of working men took extra people into the family. The estimate is that one in five of all working-class families in the latter part of the nineteenth century took in boarders in the effort to make ends meet.

For obvious reasons these women were less likely than their more prosperous contemporaries to be long lived, but for both men and women in this group the fear of a dependent old age was an ever-present fact of life. There was then no social security, no private pensions. Jane Addams has written about an Italian immigrant weeping bitterly at the death of his fourteen-year-old daughter, and when she tried to comfort him he turned to her and said, "But now who will take care of me when I can no longer work?" The industrialist who told a congressional committee that when his machines wore out he threw them out, and his workers likewise, was probably an extreme case, but it was some variation on that view which made possible the rapid industrial development of this country. I think that for workers the horrors of old age were about equal for men and women.

While the process of industrialization kept the majority of urban wage earners constantly on the edge of unemployment and disaster, for the luckier minority who shared in the newly created wealth, industrialization meant prosperity and upward social mobility. Women in such families experienced something quite new in history: time for something other than working with their hands and bearing and raising children. The demographers tell us that the birth rate began to drop in the year 1800 and that it went down steadily for the rest of the century. The combination of rising family incomes, cheap immigrant or black servants, fewer children, and the early forms of household conveniences created a new social class of women. Some turned to dress and social gatherings, big houses and fine carriages, and developed ever more refined ways of wasting time and money. Such women, in the nature of things, leave very little evidence that they have lived, and so the historian is hard put to find out much about the inner nature of their lives. If it is true, as one of my friends once remarked, that whatever you are like when you are young you will be more so when you get older—then women like these just became steadily more useless as time went by.

But there were other women who, presented with the unprecedented gift of time, began to look beyond their homes to the community, to the social problems of the industrial society, and began to organize reform groups, participate in church work, seek education, and think about their own place in the world. As early as 1797 a group of such women in New York formed a Society for the Care of Poor Widows with Young Children, setting an example that would be followed in hundreds of old and new communities for the rest of the century, of women taking responsibility through voluntary associations for what we would nowadays call welfare work. In new towns on the frontier women joined together to found churches and schools and temperance groups. In the Northeast they began to agitate for the freedom of the slaves and for better educational opportunities for themselves. By 1848 three women, veterans of the abolition movement, sent out a call to all who might be interested to meet in Seneca Falls, New York, to discuss the rights of women—and with only a few days' notice 300 people came. Once there they adopted a ringing statement, based on the Declaration of Independence, calling for an end to legal discrimination, for educational opportunity, for the right to enter the professions, and—most controversial of all—for the right to vote. American feminism was not born at Seneca Falls. It had existed here and there for a very long time, but in 1848 it came out in the open, and the Declaration of Sentiments, as it was called, provided an agenda for a women's rights movement that was to bring about some of the most pervasive social changes in the ensuing century of revolutionary social change.

Feminism was sometimes overt, as in the organized women's rights movement, but more often it was covert, as women built organizations of all sorts and created community institutions to carry out things they wanted to accomplish. Shut out, as they usually were, from traditional social structures—the bench, the bar, the medical profession, the ministry, higher education—women created their own social organizations that they themselves could run. Women doctors, denied access to male-run hospitals, built their own. A woman lawyer refused admission to the bar in Illinois and told by the Supreme Court of the United States that God did not intend her to be a lawyer, created a legal newsletter to report things lawyers need to know; it was so thoroughly well done that it soon became indispensable to male lawyers in the Middle West. Women denied admission to Harvard and Yale organized and ran Radcliffe and Bryn Mawr. Women denied the right to vote organized a political movement that after seventy years of unremitting effort wrested the suffrage from all-male Congress and all-male legislatures. Denied the right to preach, they organized the Woman's Christian Temperance Union and developed their skills in the ministry through its multiple programs. Seeing social needs, women invented solutions: kindergartens, juvenile protective associations, consumers' leagues, the Indian Rights Association, the Women's Trade Union League, the Woman's Peace Party, not to mention hundreds of local clubs with civic reform as their purpose. The voluntary association was their principle tool, and with it they changed and shaped nineteenth century America, and in the process changed and emancipated themselves.

As a fringe benefit of all this effort—none of it, I might say, easy—many women seem to have enjoyed extraordinary longevity and, what is even more important, to have remained active and effective into very old age. Evidence for this interesting fact may be found in the three-volume biographical dictionary called *Notable American Women*, which contains biographies of 1,359 women, mostly nineteenth century women, and many of the kind I have just been describing. Out of that number (nearly all were born before 1900 at a time when life expectancy was much lower than it is now), 40 percent lived to be seventy-five, and nearly 30 percent lived to be anywhere from eighty to ninety-nine.

What is even more impressive than sheer longevity—though that is impressive enough—is the fact that so many were active and effective in their chosen fields until very late in life. It would take too long to tell about each of the 364 who lived past eighty, but here are some random examples: Elizabeth Agassiz, the founder of Radcliffe, was still its president at seventy-seven; Amelia Barr, a novelist, wrote her last novel when she was eighty-seven; Lenora Barry, who organized women for the Knights of Labor, was still making public speeches at seventy-eight; Clara Barton, the founder of the Red Cross, was at her desk when she was ninety and was said to be still "vigorous and of youthful appearance." Alva Belmont, suffragist, at seventy-seven appeared before an international gathering to urge the removal of legal disabilities against women. Joanna Bethune, daughter of the woman who founded that first Society for the Care of Poor Widows with Young Children, was still active in the affairs of an Orphan Asylum at ninety. Elizabeth Blackwell, one of the first woman doctors, practiced medicine until she was seventy-four and continued active for ten years after that. Her sister-in-law Antoinette Brown Blackwell, suffragist and minister, gave her last public lecture at the age of ninety.

In other words, feminism—which I think of as women standing on their own feet and acting in any sphere of life where there is important work to be done—is one of the few effective antidotes to aging we have yet discovered. Being an independent woman with a purpose in life does not provide immortality, of course, but it certainly seems to promote longevity and, what is more important, seems to be the best way to experience a useful and interesting old age.

I suppose there are some statisticians and demographers who are ready to take issue with my evidence and to offer other possible explanations for the longevity represented in this particular group of women, but the more one studies the biographies themselves, the more the explanation seems valid. There is, I would argue, a strong relationship between the willingness of these women to commit themselves to serious tasks and hard work, and the nature of their aging.

In the course of writing a biography for a forthcoming supplement to *Notable American Women,* I stumbled on what might almost be called a laboratory experiment bearing on this question. Probably no state in the union was less open to the idea of woman suffrage in the 1880s than the state of Mississippi, but a woman living in Greenville, a leader in her church and in the Women's Christian Temperance Union, thought women should vote, and so she organized, in spite of considerable social disapproval, the Mississippi Suffrage Association. She was a born politician. Even though she could not vote, she became one of the two leaders of the Democratic party in her county, and when the Nineteenth Amendment passed, she, at age sixty-one, was the first woman elected to the Mississippi legislature. There she developed an outstanding record; among other things, a committee she chaired reorganized the administration of welfare institutions in the state. In 1924, in her mid-sixties, she represented Mississippi at the Democratic Convention and attracted considerable national attention for the leadership she exerted there.

Her life went on in this vein until, at seventy-three, she began to develop cataracts, and in her usual way of taking life head-on, she left Greenville, which had always been her home, and built a little house next door to her son who lived in another town. In a few months her children were startled to see their mother begin to grow old, to lose interest in life. Fortunately, one daughter diagnosed the problem at once and urged her mother to return to Greenville where—as she herself had put it—she could always stir something up by just walking down the street. Sure enough, back in the milieu of her active political life, she shed her aging ways. She found a doctor who cured the cataracts without an operation. Sixteen years later she was still teaching a popular Sunday School class, making public addresses, writing interesting letters, and managing her own money so skillfully that though she had had only a modest inheritance she was able, when she died at eighty-nine, to leave her children a substantial legacy. The only regrettable part of this story is that in 1948 with her usual skill Mrs. Somerville supported Strom Thurmond's States' Rights party, and of course with that kind of skill at his disposal, he carried the state.

One could go on and on, but it is time to turn to the final point: Are there lessons in all this history that bear upon our own problems, those which I set forth at the beginning? Let me take them up in reverse order.

First, when women outnumber men in large numbers, the importance of being an independent woman is obvious. If one must expect to live for some significant part of life as a widow, it is important to have one's own identity and one's own work. If a woman has always been defined as somebody's wife or somebody's mother, she is not in very good shape at age sixty-five to become a person in her own right. Furthermore, if one is likely to live till eighty or ninety, it is exceedingly important to have a great deal of unfinished work on hand to make it worth getting up in the morning. While some few of us are designed for the contemplative life, many more are most alive when most involved with real problems beyond their own daily existence.

Perhaps therefore it is fortunate that the growing size of the aging population provides just such a set of social needs as historically have called forth the best in women. We are inundated with statistics about the problems of older people and by demands that the government or the foundations or somebody do something about them. Without denying the importance of things the government should and must do, perhaps we should begin to look in a different direction. Just as a substantial number of Americans have turned their backs on the seemingly endless debates in Congress over an energy policy, and have begun to put on sweaters, build greenhouses, polish up their bicycles, create van pools, invest in new kinds of woodstoves, and turn out the lights, just so I would suggest that it is time for those of us who are passing those magic deadlines of sixty or seventy—or one hundred for that matter—to turn our attention to what we ourselves can do for the aging population to which we belong. At most the government can make sure that old people have enough to eat and adequate medical care, but beyond that it cannot in the very nature of things meet all the thousand-and-one other needs which older people share. On the other hand, the list of do-it-yourself possibilities is long.

We have hardly scratched the surface in community cooperation, for example. No individual can solve the problem of rising energy costs, but communal experiments may help. Some of our children have demonstrated how much can be done to cut loose from the money economy and yet live a good life. I wonder how many of us have the courage to follow their example?

Because in this society women are healthier and live longer than men, and also because their whole history shows that they have been exceedingly good at forming voluntary associations to meet social needs, it seems obvious to me that the next step is for older women themselves to take the lead in organizing to meet some of these well-identified needs. I think it was a woman who coined the slogan, "Don't agonize, organize."

Discrimination against the aged is a complex phenomenon, part of which rests on age-old stereotypes and prejudices, but some of it is a reflection of fear, fear that the increasing numbers of older people will become an intolerable burden on the young. The eighteenth century has something to tell us on this score: useful people are respected no matter how old they are. There are so many things to be done in this society that there is no need for anyone to become old from simple lack of useful work to do. If more people believed this and acted on it, I think the problem of discrimination against the aged would diminish considerably.

Furthermore, there is the great incentive, the fringe benefit of what serious undertakings outside one's own personal life can do for the person. Our nineteenth century forbears are witness to this: when the society seemed forbidding, saying, "Because you are a woman, you can't do that," they took their own initiatives, created their own groups, and in the process found themselves developing into healthy, long-lived, and interesting people. Just so, I would argue, when someone says, "You're too old to do that," the response must be: "Who says so?"

Such attitudes have been held by women for a long time. For several years two quotations have hung over my desk. One comes from a letter written by that extraordinary suffragist Elizabeth Cady Stanton to her close friend and collaborator Susan B. Anthony. Stanton had just given birth to her sixth child, and Anthony, who was single, had complained about the way numerous babies were delaying their mother's work for suffrage. "Courage, Susan," Stanton wrote, "We shall not reach our prime before fifty and then we shall have twenty good years at least." Her expectation, as it turned out, was too modest; they lived to be eighty-two and eighty-three, respectively, each working to the last day of her life.

The other quotation is from a letter written to Julia Ward Howe (an all-purpose activist through her ninety-three years) by an older aunt when Howe herself was approaching middle age. "Julia!" the aunt wrote with appropriate exclamation marks, "Never grow old. Whenever you think you cannot do something, get up and do it."

Both these women understood what I have been restating here: the process of aging is to a large extent a self-fulfilling prophecy. If one expects to grow feeble and dull and to be scorned by the young, it is very likely to happen. If one is, like the women I have been describing, too busy even to think much about aging, the process in some mysterious way seems to slow down and to be less debilitating than among people whose minds are on themselves.

I have been talking mainly about women, but clearly the underlying thesis is not tied to sex. All of us, like Tennyson's Ulysses, know in our hearts that it's dull to "pause, to make an end, /To rust unburnished, not to shine in use!/As though to breathe were life!" And so Ulysses called his friends, his shipmates, to a cooperative endeavor: "'is not too late to seek a newer world/Push off, and sitting well in order smite/The sounding furrows."

If we too can push off, even in new directions, perhaps some historian of the future will be writing that in the last decades of the twentieth century, the United States of America developed a new élan, not in spite of, but because of, its aging population.

REFERENCES

Biddle, G.B., and S.D. Lowrie. 1942. "Susanna Wright." In *Notable Pennsylvania Women*. Philadelphia: University of Pennsylvania Press.

Demos, John. 1978. "Old Age in Early New England." In *Turning Points*, edited by John Demos and S.S. Bocock. Chicago: University of Chicago Press.

Drinker, Elizabeth. 1797. Unpublished journal, Historical Society of Pennsylvania.

Freeman, Mary E. Wilkins. 1899. *In Colonial Times*. Boston: Lathrop and Co.

James, Edward, and Janet James, eds. 1971. *Notable American Women*. Cambridge, Mass.: Harvard University Press.

Keyssar, Alexander. 1974. "Widowhood in Eighteenth Century Massachusetts: A Problem in the History of the Family." *Perspectives* 7:83–119.

Mathis, Ray, ed. 1979. *John Horry Den: South Carolina Aristocrat on the Alabama Frontier*. University, Alabama: University of Alabama Press.

Van Doren, Carl, ed. 1950. *The Letters of Benjamin Franklin and Jane Mecom*. Princeton: Princeton University Press.

UNIVERSITY OF MICHIGAN CREATIVITY AND AGING

INTRODUCTION

Harold R. Johnson and Beth Spencer

Aging is viewed far too frequently as an unproductive and un-satisfying stage of the life cycle. Thus, when we were pre-sented with an opportunity to offer a lecture series in 1980, we quickly settled on the theme of creativity and aging. This seemed an ideal occasion to continue our efforts to celebrate artists in their later years and to have scholars, as well as the artists themselves, reflect on the relationship between creativi-ty and aging.

We hoped that by weaving together artistic performances and scholarly presentations, we would draw broader audiences than those generally attracted to gerontological lectures. This proved to be the case. Each week the auditorium was filled with different groups of people: young and old students and scholars of the arts and sciences; busloads of older people from social clubs, senior housing complexes, and nutrition sites; many generations of blues lovers; women's groups; poetry lov-ers; and folk music aficionados for the final event. It is our be-lief that this wide range of people joined in our celebration of the creativity so vividly demonstrated by the artists and speakers in our series. It is our hope that they left with a clearer vision of the creative potential across the life span and a renewed inspiration for their own old age.

In later years, as at all ages, creativity is manifested in many ways. Too often we tend to separate creativity in the later years into basket-weaving types of activities on the one hand, or the work of Picasso, Matisse, and other long-lived creators whose names are always paraded out, on the other. But an enormous spectrum of creative activity lies between these extremes. There are those who have devoted their lives to the process of creation—as scientist, mathematician, poet, or scholar—who continue doing what they have always done in old age. Many other people have the opportunity for the first time in retirement to devote hours to the pursuit of creative activities. Still others return in their later years to artistic endeavors of their youth that were abandoned during middle age.

In choosing the artists and speakers for our creativity and aging series, we tried to find individuals whose lives represented different approaches to creativity. It quickly became clear that our problem was not finding outstanding performers and scholars who were older, but rather limiting ourselves to only a few of the many possibilities. Our aim was to find people who could help us explore the complex interrelationship between creativity and aging: how attitudes toward, and experiences of, aging enhance, alter, or require modifications of the creative process; and conversely, how creativity enriches the experience of aging.

The four chapters in this part do indeed explore this relationship from very different artistic and disciplinary vantage points. They stand well on their own, but two were greatly enhanced by the musical performances that accompanied them.

When we were considering a keynote speaker for the creativity and aging series—someone who could provide a foundation and framework for the rest of the events—Dr. John A.B. McLeish was an obvious choice. His 1976 book, *The Ulyssean Adult: Creativity in the Middle and Later Years*, is regarded as a seminal work in the area of adult creativity.

In his paper Dr. McLeish eloquently discusses selected definitions of creativity and some of the myths about the creative process, particularly as they apply to the older creator. He points out some of the characteristics of the creative individual, providing many examples and anecdotes from his research experiences, and reflects on conditions that may inhibit creativity among older people. Finally, he offers suggestions to people who may be concerned with nurturing their own creative urges.

The second event in the series was a talk and poetry reading by May Sarton, the noted American poet, novelist, and chronicler, who shared some of her thoughts about how her own aging is affecting her writing and her life as a writer. The poems she chose to include are celebrations of old people whom she has known, words of praise for the old and of thanks to those who inspired and encouraged her.

The third event featured a talk by Professor James A. Standifer and a performance by Sippie Wallace, a blues singer in her eighties who has recently returned to the stage. Ms. Wallace's superbly sensuous stage presence and the vitality of her singing performance captivated the audience and brought to life many of the issues discussed by Dr. Standifer in his authoritative chapter on elderly black blues and jazz musicians.

In the past two years, Dr. Standifer has traveled all over the world talking with older black musicians and singers about their early experiences in the entertainment world. During these interviews, he also talked with many of the artists about how their musicianship has improved or changed with increasing age, what accommodations they have made because of age, and how the fact of being an artist has affected their later lives. Dr. Standifer's chapter includes some of the responses to these questions about creativity and aging and his reflections on this relationship, particularly for nonclassical black performers.

For the final event of the series, it was our privilege to bring Dr. Alan Jabbour, director of the American Folklife Center at the Library of Congress, to Ann Arbor. His informative and entertaining talk was followed by two performing groups: the Sinclair Trio and the Mainers.

The Sinclair Trio, a folk music group from Sheridan, Michigan, is composed of three men who began performing together in retirement on instruments they had played in their youths. The Sinclair brothers harmonize on homemade hammer dulcimers, accompanied by Ken Staines on banjo, ukelele, mandolin, or autoharp. Their great enthusiasm and lively music quickly had the audience clapping and foot stomping. The second group, a husband-wife team, are often joined on stage by their son. Wade Mainer, who was part of the original Mainer Mountaineers of North Carolina in the 1930s and 1940s, gave up professional singing and worked in an auto plant for many years. Since retiring he and his wife have returned to the stage, appearing at folk concerts all over the country.

These groups are part of a nationwide revival in public interest in folk arts and crafts. Little attention has yet been paid to the remarkable predominance of older adults working as artists in this area. This may be due in part to the limited academic interest in folk artists themselves; and it also results from the tendency of most folk artists to work and live away from the public eye.

Many strains of Dr. McLeish's discussion of creativity are picked up again by Dr. Jabbour, but this time from the perspective of a folklorist and superb storyteller. Dr. Jabbour's stories and penetrating insights provide a thoughtful ending to the series and leave us with many questions for future investigations of creativity and aging. His example of the life rhythms of creativity among fiddlers is a fascinating account, reminiscent of a pattern discerned by Dr. Standifer among many of the blues and jazz artists he interviewed. In a very personal way, Dr. Jabbour is able to bring to life the intergenerational bonds fostered by creativity and to articulate the fundamental importance of cultural exchange among the old and the young.

The Institute of Gerontology is very grateful for having had the opportunity to focus the attention of the public on some of the more positive aspects of aging through the creativity and aging series. Over the years we have devoted considerable time and attention to dispelling the notion that aging is primarily an experience of ever-multiplying problems. Often this problem-centered orientation—which is a very relative and culture-bound perspective—has dominated the field of gerontology to the exclusion of more positive ways of thinking about aging and the aged. We have attempted to combat ageism by placing a greater emphasis on research and on the humanities, through the development of courses and bibliographies, and by encouraging scholars from the humanities to become interested in aging. Projects such as *Images of Old Age in America,*

1790 –1977, a book and traveling visual essay, and the aging and the art of living symposium held at the University of Michigan a few years ago have contributed toward providing broader and more positive perspectives on aging. It is our hope that this series has also helped to change some negative attitudes toward growing old and has inspired some people in their efforts to be creative.

Although there are too many people who worked very hard planning the creativity and aging series and bringing it to fruition to thank each individually, special appreciation and thanks must go to Professor Dorothy Coons, Eloise Snyder, Carol Hollenshead, and Donna Goodrid for their leadership and untiring efforts to make it a great success.

5 THE CONTINUUM OF CREATIVITY

John A.B. McLeish

In considering creativity in the later years, we have the satisfaction of knowing that we are dealing with a sublime topic. Nothing can be of more concern to the human species than creativity, and no subject can be more valuable for inquiry in our time than the creative potential of older adults.

A review of research and literature during the past thirty years uncovers a variety of issues and insights that illuminate the creative functioning and potentialities of the later adult years, often in very different ways. For example, to Eric Fromm (1959) creativity is not so much *doing* something as *being* something: "Creativity is the ability *to see* (or to be *aware*) and *to respond*" (p. 44). To Carl Rogers (1959), creativity is "the emergence in action of a novel product, growing out of the uniqueness of the individual on the one hand, and the materials, events, people, or circumstances of his life on the other" (p. 71). Thus Rogers felt that creativity meant delivering an observable product, though that product might be so unrecognized as reforming one's own personality through psychotherapy. Dorothy Sayers's views disagreed: one could be, Sayers remarked, a poet without writing a poem—a useful insight but one perilous for many lazy would-be creators.

The creative process fascinated Abraham Maslow (1959), who separated creativity into two types: first, "special talent creativity"—the creativity of the gifted inventor, scientist, poet, sculptor, architect, novelist, and so on; and second, "self-actualizing creativeness," which Maslow defined as showing itself much more in creative changes in the personality, and in a tendency to do anything creatively—that is, *living* creatively.

In J.W. Haefele's fine and much-neglected work, *Creativity and Innovation* (1962) occurs this definition: the creative thing or act "is a new combination formed from pieces already in the mind by symbolic manipulation during dissociated thought" (p. 5). And Haefele, by profession an industrial chemist, adds, "It is the same in arts as in science" (p. 5).

Commentators as casual as John W. Gardner (1964), and as scholarly as Silvano Arieti (1976), both agree that some potential for creativity is found in all human beings, and they note the enormous range of the process through higher and lower levels. Arieti is especially interesting with his careful distinctions among spontaneity, originality, and creativity. He remarks: "Man's spontaneity and originality manifest themselves in a flow of images, feelings, and ideas. [But] if the average person does little or nothing with these free images and ideas—if he only experiences them . . . he cannot be considered creative" (p. 7). Arieti believes that "a person may lose originality and retain spontaneity in the process of growing up and becoming educated" (p. 7). But he also remarks that an individual may later "become original again," even though to do so "he must use different ways, and the new forms of originality will be at least partially derivative" (p. 8).

For this chapter, I add one further definition of creativity: Creativity is the process by which a person employs both conscious and unconscious domains of the mind to combine various existing materials into fresh constructions or configurations that, in some degree, cause significant changes in the self-system of the person concerned, or significantly alter the environment surrounding the person, whether such a change is great or small.

Another way of considering the meaning of creativity is by seeking to identify what appear to be typical traits of men and women clearly employing their talents in productive ways. Resources for this investigation can be found in many biographies of people in the arts, inventors, statesmen, scientists, and others; in the many anonymous reports of psychotherapists interested in the creative process; and in the lives of private men and women.

Surveying part of the evidence, John Gardner (1964) lists four major traits: (1) openness to fresh experiences, (2) independence, (3) flexibility, and (4) order—by which he means the capacity to discipline oneself sufficiently to harness and use the flow of images, feelings, and ideas. Frank Barron (1963), whose work on creativity and psychological health remains seminal, was fascinated by the role of independence in creative achievement; he speaks regretfully of those men and women who have become "yielders" to suffocating environments.

Calvin Taylor and J. Holland, in an important study (1964) of possible predictors of creative performance, observe:

> There is some evidence that creative persons are more autonomous than others, more self-sufficient, more independent in judgment, more open to the irrational in themselves, more stable, more feminine in interests and characteristics (especially in awareness of their impulses), more dominant and self-assertive, more complex, more self-accepting, more resourceful and adventurous, more radical (the old word was Bohemian), more self-controlled, possibly more emotionally sensitive, more introverted but also more bold (pp. 27–28).

Possible amendments to these listed traits, of course, rise in clouds. One is the warning that we should rather speak of "most creative" and "more creative" persons, rather than suggesting categories of people simply creative or noncreative. Still, the list is rich in applicability to great numbers of creative people, and may help fill in a backdrop for my own references to creativity and aging.

How far is intelligence a factor in creativity? Many of us would accept Haefele's dictum (1962): "A creator must be intelligent, but even a highly intelligent person is not necessarily creative" (pp. 116ff.), although the range of creative activity is so great and the definition of intelligence so complex that even this useful statement has to be accepted with reservations.

When L.M. Terman reported after thirty-four years on the life progress of his 1,000 "gifted children" (a term I have always disliked), he was able to show many to have been successful but few highly creative. However, we have much to learn yet about the manifestations of creativity in private lives and also about the validity of criteria in formally testing creative powers.

The fascinating question also arises as to whether some forms of intelligence are not actual blocks to creative achievement. This question emerges in the scenes described by Edward de Bono (1967) where so-called "vertical thinkers," as he calls the people highly programmed into exactly logical thinking, are frequently inhibited from creative solutions that they might reach through "lateral" (essentially divergent) thinking. Incidentally, even here, in the domain where Jerome Bruner has also written about the importance of guessing, the mandated phrase that immediately follows is *"intelligent* guessing." Or again, in certain of the arts, if we accept Simone de Beauvoir's insistence that there is an indispensable link between warm sexual feeling and creativity, is it fair to ask whether the cold intelligence, however "high," is an inhibitor of creativity?

In his 1968 study, *Human Intelligence*, H.J. Butcher says of creativity that "it implies a high degree of ability at divergent-type thinking (probably allied to a particular kind of temperament and motivation), enabling us to reserve 'intelligence' as a description of the convergent thinking exemplified in the education of relations and correlates (in Spearman's language)" (p. 97). Although such a dichotomy has value, I am myself more drawn to the lonely voice of Stanley Burnshaw, writing in *The Seamless Web* (1970): "The old conscious/unconscious dichotomy is crude. The mind is, after all, all one mind, however unlike its manifestations, however various its capacities, to compose, dissect, choose, wander, concentrate, and so on. For the poet, for example, composition must be an act of their collaboration" (p. 72). Such a holistic cry must at least be heard in a discussion like this.[1]

---

1. The other dichotomy, the "left brain/right brain" role in creativity is usefully discussed in Restak (1979).

What are the environments in which creativity seems to flourish or wilt? C.K. Tuska (1955) once interestingly defined creativity in terms of an equation: "Favorable circumstances *plus* exercise or creative imagination *times* effort to the nth power *plus* good luck *equals* the creative product" (see pp. 93–98). But what are the favorable circumstances?

Arieti (1976) suggests—as do I—that although "creativity may occur at any age in life, it seems logical to assume (although it is by no means certain) that an inclination toward creativity must be fostered in childhood and/or adolescence" (pp. 36–62). If so, the role of the family in helping foster early creativity should be crucial, and seemingly in many cases it is, for better or for worse. Will the home environment, in John Gardner's (1964) useful phrase, "smother or release" the creative impulses of children? No doubt in numerous cases the power of the creative talent will break through, regardless of environment. This is well symbolized in the story of Alexander the Great visiting Diogenes and asking whether he could do anything for the famous scientist; Diogenes replied, "Just stand out of my light." [2]

But one study (Getzel and Jackson 1962) has shown that the attitudes of parents, for example, seem to matter substantially: whether, negatively, they surround their children by overcontrol, inhibiting anxieties, worries that seemingly unusual children may be or appear odd, impractical, introverted, ill equipped for the race to the social conventionalities of success. Or whether, affirmatively, parents facilitate creativity by permitting individual divergence and accepting risks.

The school is obviously the other great social agency that may help release or inhibit creative potentials, and here we are especially indebted to the extensive studies of E. Paul Torrance (1963). Not surprisingly, in the light of what has been said before, Torrance was able to identify richly facilitative school environments for children as those where the teachers gave "time-out" from evaluated performances, treated the ideas of children with respect—especially their unusual

---

2. However, Thomas Gray's poignant phrase from the *Elegy* also resounds in one's mind: "mute inglorious Miltons."

ideas—and took care to see that self-initiated learning was encouraged and rewarded.

It is a fascinating question for those of us chiefly interested in creativity and aging to consider whether today's older adults were especially affected by the attitudes of schools and teachers in classroom settings where Torrance's desired conditions were often blocked by rigidly structured curricula and pedagogic dogmatism.

The noted Goethe scholar Barker Fairley, still painting with imaginative power and exhibiting at age ninety-three in Toronto, has told me that from age seven until age forty-five when he was finally induced to join a weekend sketching party, he abstained from painting because he had been told at school that he had no talent. I am sure that many others could give comparable experiences, so sensitive are many children to what seems to be the authoritative voice of the adult in the realm of talent. What might be termed *manifest talent* probably frequently is recognized and encouraged; it is the fragile, tentative, slowly developing talent that is likely to be overlooked or inhibited. One must at once add, however, that the autobiographies of many creative people and many of our own lives have been marked by the rich stimulus provided by interested mentors and teachers.

One of the curiosities of educational systems across the years has been their failure to study and specifically facilitate the creative process as such. Haefele (1962) remarks: "Eighteen years in school exercised the learning faculty, the memory faculty, the reasoning faculty, the verbal reconstruction for the teacher faculty—everything but the creative faculty: there wasn't time for that" (p. 116ff.). Haefele was in his mature years when he wrote that, and again we confront a phenomenon about the environments of creativity which is especially applicable to middle-aged and older adults.

Does middle- and later-life creativity in fact resonate from early life experiences? Of course it does. However, continuing or resumed creative production, or wholly new production in later life, is closely connected with the individual adult's motivational system, changing self-image, and mental and emotional health. Later creativity is also promoted for some and inhibited for others by turbulent intersections of the life journey; and we who voyage later in life also confront formidable constraints of time, energy, resources, and triumphs and failures of the will.

What motivates the human adult in any case to create? To Arthur Koestler (1969), "Every adult is a holon, and feels the need to be part of something that transcends the narrow boundaries of the self... the magic of form... the ocean of sound, or the mathematical symbols of convergence in the infinite" (p. 190). To John Milton in *Lycidas*, the desire to be famous is a frequent motive: "Fame is the spur that the clear spirit doth raise,/.../To scorn delights and live laborious days." Haefele talks more simply about "the human need for recognition," while Lawrence Cranberg, on the other hand, warns of the perils of *over*-recognition in *extinguishing* motivation, as in the case of Isaac Newton.

Many men and women, notably in their middle and later years, feel the need to engage in some form of creativity in dozens of possible channels, in order directly or indirectly to change their own lives and selves. This is what Yeats meant when he wrote:

> The friends that have it I do wrong
> Whenever I remake a song,
> Should know what issue is at stake:
> It is myself that I remake.

And this is likewise what the noted Canadian painter Arthur Lismer meant by an offhand remark to me when I was assembling the data for his biography: "That great work of art, John—one's own life."

So convinced was Abraham Maslow (1959) of the basic thrust of this self-actualizing creativeness that he wrote: "If there were no choking-off forces, we might expect that every human being would show this special type of creativity" (p. 85). It is true; yet I think we must not fail to remind ourselves that great numbers of human beings also engage in some creative activity because it is fun—they feel joyful doing so.

The demands of the market have themselves been sufficient to spur some creative people into activity, and also to lead to significant alterations in the creative course. Handel's fame as a writer of oratorios might never have been born had it not been for his conviction in his mature career that his opera market had been lost to new forms from Italy. The loss of Sir Walter Scott's market as a poet preceded his finding again the half-finished manuscript of *Waverley*, begun nine years earlier, and his embarking on a career as novelist. The reverse was true of Thomas Hardy: his disgust at the critical reception of his splendid novels led him to embark at nearly sixty upon a career exclusively as poet—a career yielding thirty years of undiminished power. One could write a whole chapter alone on these changes caused by new motives, and this would include in our time the fascinating subject of creative life changes leading to second, third, and fourth careers.

Encouragement from others significant in one's life is often a powerful motivator. The life histories of creative men and women are filled with contributions of what I call "offstage" people—the usually unknown and therefore uncelebrated encouragers and facilitators of creative people and actions. A few are themselves famous: Goethe's Duke of Weimar, Mozart's difficult archbishop, and others; but in general the offstage people are likely to resemble Agnes de Mille's devoted and selfless mother, and like her, they often miss the ultimate acclaim of the beloved person they helped on. There are also, of course, offstage discouragers who have played a somber and destructive role—like the mistress of Andrea del Sarto, at least as Browning saw her; the rejecting lover of Rudolph Zimmer; or cold and discouraging employers; and insensitive and even vicious critics. But the role of offstage encouragers and discouragers remains a tantalizing topic in creativity.

Sometimes the encourager has been the state or some foundation, agency, or commissioning corporation—this series is itself an example. Whatever the source, the role of encouragement in motivating others to begin or to resume creative acts in a high one. We are used to hearing how the young need encouragement. When will we hear more and see more of encouragement for the old?

What is it, in fact, that causes men and women in their middle and later years to abandon personal creative activity, or to refuse to resume it when the chances offer? What causes them to live lives of low creative candlepower—whether lives other-

wise good and in certain ways admirable or desolate and destructive—rather than to seek and risk personal creative
adventures?

Humanistic psychology and psychotherapy provide one interesting answer, by suggesting that one major obstruction
can be the self-image (see Horney 1950; Adler 1965; and Arieti 1976). In early youth, for a variety of reasons, many potentially creative people construct a grandiose image of
themselves for the future, an image usually secret but for a
time assiduously cultivated. When the time fails to fulfill
these expectations—when dreams of grandeur dissolve—then
in many cases the adult, now mature in years but not necessarily in judgment, simply abandons the field. And this is a
great pity.

Sometimes the early promise is unfulfilled for the tragic reason that although there is an abundance of talent, certain negative forces in the self-system or the life scenario thwart its
development. This situation is vividly illustrated by the noted
British critic Cyril Connolly in his memoir, significantly entitled *Enemies of Promise* (1970). Connolly reminds us that talent can be dispersed or stifled by the involvement of the
creative person in other negative life activities that drain energies and lower creative tone, including addictions and mal-
functions of the spirit.

A persistent legend in ideas about creativity in the arts is
that neurosis is beneficial. Shakespeare may have reinforced
this myth when he wrote in *A Midsummer Night's Dream*:
"The lunatic, the lover, and the poet/Are of imagination all
compact." Even so, whatever expert evidence we can assemble
indicates that neurosis is a block rather than an aid to the creative process. It is true that R.B. Cattell's study of highly creative scientists found an unusually high level of anxiety
(including irritability and excitability) in these men; but Cattell made a great distinction between this form of anxiety and
neurosis, and concluded that overt neurotic disorder was relatively rare among them. In the arts, Barron's study, *Creativity
and Psychological Health* (1963), makes the important point
that one distinction between the effectively creative person
and the neurotic individual is that the former is able to use the
exercise of regressing into the fantastic world of the uncon-

scious to achieve his creative purpose but then emerges, not being trapped there like the neurotic.

Nonetheless, I have always felt the position of commentators like L.S. Kubie (1958) and Arthur Koestler (1969) to be extreme: that neurosis is always antithetical to creative production. I differentiate between what one might term "conventional" or "operable" neurosis and clinical or disabling neurosis. For example, I have no doubt that fear of heights and closed spaces and of spiders and snakes is neurotic. But these are the kinds of conventional neurotic feelings that strike me as insight makers and compassion makers, and at least in the arts and in Maslow's "interpersonal creativity," these feelings may be enablers of the creative spirit. Whatever helps us share the fears and sorrows of the great suffering, laughing, aspiring species to which we belong seems to me contributive. However, disabling neurosis is another matter, although even here certain creative functions may emerge.

Of one thing we may be sure: it is not good for the human spirit to keep on for months and years contemplating personal creative adventures that are never actualized. William Blake once wrote: "Energy is Eternal Delight: he who desires but acts not, breeds pestilence." Dorothy Sayers had another term: "The energy turns demonic." Such dramatic fates may not be one's lot in leaving unused the potentialities of one's special gifts. But something uncomfortably like them may occur; and at the least one will miss a great affirmative experience in one's life: the power of creative activity in healing the stresses, sorrows, and loneliness encountered on the life journey.[3]

Perhaps the greatest inhibitors of successful creativity in the later middle years and beyond are *the myths of aging*. I have dealt with these at great length in *The Ulyssean Adult* (1976) and in subsequent papers, and here I wish merely to cite them and to draw attention to two that are specially relevant. The five major myths are: (1) the myth of inevitable senility; (2) the myth of inevitable sexual impotence; (3) the myth of inevitable rigidifying of attitudes and opinions; (4) the

---

3. On the other hand, a strong soul long prevented by circumstances from beginning its creative exploit may even gain strength from secretly keeping the flame. A remarkable case in point is the modern black naive painter, Clementine Hunter.

myth of inevitable decline of learning powers; (5) the myth of inevitable loss of creative powers and production. Only the last two are highly relevant to my present theme. The urge to learn, as described by Cyril Houle in a small, beautiful study, *The Inquiring Mind* (1961), and again in Ronald Gross's admirable book, *The Lifelong Learner* (1977), has qualities so close to those I have already suggested for the urge to create, that it is fair to consider both together in rejecting most of the negative myths about learning and creating.

In the case of human learning, there is now mounting evidence that later-age adults with viable health and strong motivation retain firepower enough for a very long sequence of rich and varied learning adventures (see K.W. Schaie; Gordon Blum; Carl Eisdorfer; A.S. Friedman; S. Granick; L.F. Jarvik; H. McCluskey; and I. Lorge). The word "enough" is crucial. We have for too long been deluded by the mesmerized attention given by certain researchers to timed performances—an attitude perhaps typical of our "instamatic" society. It is not the timed performance but the ultimate quality of the learning performance that should concern us. The same is true of creative exploits. The fact that the British novelist M.M. Kaye took most of a decade from her middle sixties into her early seventies to complete her 1,000-page novel *The Far Pavilions* (1975), fighting cancer successfully along the way, takes nothing from the quality of the performance.

The myth that creative power reaches some kind of life peak in the thirties of the life journey and then steadily descends was furthered in a 1953 study by H.C. Lehman, *Age and Achievement*. Yet its numerous erroneous conclusions are still being reproduced in some recent popular books as though coming on tablets of stone. In fact, in spite of all the statistical busywork put into the Lehman thesis, his conclusions on the peaking of creative power in the arts are simply grotesque. In her massive work, *The Coming of Age* (1972), Simone de Beauvoir properly dismisses Lehman and associates with a terse footnote, although she admits that there may be something to the Lehman claims in the sphere of scientific discovery. On the other hand, various studies have shown the extended creativity of well-known scientists across the life span (see Roe 1952); and in a small but thorough review that I made in 1975, I had no trouble identifying 125 noted scientists from all fields who were incontestably richly creative into their late, even very late years (see McLeish 1976, pp. 287–287).

The fallacy of the whole Lehman approach even here was to assume that creative staying power could be handily assessed by locating the life dates of alleged masterpiece performances. Any investigation of the sustained creativity of any man or woman should be based on an examination of the whole working and creating life, and this presents quite a different scenario. A splendid example among many is A. Vibert Douglas's comment (1956) in her life of the astrophysicist A.S. Eddington. Noting that Eddington did not lose his rich creativity through his fifties and early sixties (he died at sixty-two), Douglas writes of his posthumously published study, *Fundamental Theory:* "It was an unfinished symphony standing as a challenge to the musicians among natural philosophers of the future." Eddington is one example among many of my own contention elsewhere (1976): "A scientist may show brilliant creative power in the assault upon some most formidable problem without taking the bastion" (p. 152).

There is, in fact, no good theoretical reason why human creativity should not be richly maintained across the life journey. Those who continue to talk vaguely about the decline of powers should be less vague: What powers are they talking about?

To the extent that creativity involves the play of the conscious mind, it is evident enough that there are rich resources in our continuing capacity to learn. Wilma Donahue's (1975) judgment is substantially true: "Cerebral function is the most dependable servant that can be called upon over a long span of years." At eighty Donahue illustrates her own contention as she directs the International Institute for Social Gerontology in Washington, D.C.

To the extent that creativity involves the play of the unconscious mind, what is the rationale that could suggest that this beautiful and mysterious reservoir of fantasy and association is shallower in the later years, with all their additional inputs of experience? Nor is there evidence that the strange domain of the preconscious, the unverbalized twilight zone of creativity, is somehow affected negatively by the passing years.

Neither does Berne's "OK Child" need to disappear—that child-self who symbolizes the sense of wonder toward life, of search and curiosity, of openness to the fun and absurdity of life; nor need he fall sadly silent in the daily lives and thoughts of great numbers of people in their later years. And if he sleeps, we have evidence that he can be awakened.

Thus we come to the crux of the matter. It is not the creative powers that decline and die. What may and do decline, also in huge numbers of older adults, are the will to create, the confidence that they can still create, the summoning up of physical and psychic energy, the stamina to continue through difficulties, and the continuous readiness to change: to refresh and renew the mind and the innermost self that otherwise will be left stagnant by the bitterness of former failures, endlessly replayed, and by destructive sorrows, or by former sins, real or imagined. Without the warm and loving alliance of the whole psyche, the creative powers cannot be richly released.

For the student of the creative process, the creator is just as interesting as the product, however excellent. This closing section will therefore survey some of the attitudes of about 200 creative people, who might be termed publicly known creators, and about thirty private men and women whom I queried for the purpose of this chapter. My concentration from here on is wholly on creativity as seen in action from the later middle years to the very late years.

The first striking fact about these people is how dissimilar they are. They come from a very wide spectrum of creative arenas—the arts, statecraft, invention, science, personal relations, with the predominance in the various lively arts. These creative men and women come from widely varied backgrounds; they are of every physical type; they have had widely different personal lives; and their work and play habits are also a kaleidoscope of interests and styles. In addition, their involvement in their careers often differs. Many—notably, scientists and painters—extend a continuous career in a single creative arena from youth to very late life; many find a new major creative channel in middle age or even very late age; and many begin, then suspend activity for many years, then return to it or to a closely associated field. Some, of course, simultaneously operate in two or more creative fields;

and some use one field to stimulate another—for example, music to facilitate writing.

However, the equally striking fact about these creators, public and private (even obscure), is how similar they are in traits and practices of the creative life. For one thing, these people possess a life-giving and life-loving force which perhaps can best be called "exuberance." This quality is seen in its most exotic form in the fervor and gaiety of the great black musical performers; it is magnetically and joyously present, for example, in a creative jazz performer of advanced years like Alberta Hunter or Eubie Blake.[4] It is found in a quieter but still marked degree in a Henry Miller, a Picasso, a Jonas Salk, a James Baldwin, a Buckminster Fuller, a Martha Graham, a Le Corbusier, a Pierre Trudeau, and innumerable others. However quietly the rheostat of creative exuberance may be lowered according to the public face of the creator, a typical presence in the personality is this enthusiasm of the spirit, regardless of the inevitable setbacks and passing sorrows of the creative experience.

Where does this exuberance, which is typically sustained to the end of the life journey, come from? Partly, no doubt, from the genes; but much of it clearly derives from a feeling of long-held or acquired joy in having taken a role, however known or unknown to the world, in the pageant of the cosmos.

Another common trait among creative people is a marked tenacity, often requiring a dogged courage in carrying through the creative project to its conclusion. This is notable in certain scientific experimenters and in invention, where the creative adult will perhaps return not dozens but hundreds of times to try to solve the enigma; or, as Robert Frost once put it when speaking about completing a difficult poem, to experiment until "the box clicks shut."

Once again, one thinks with a certain awe of M.M. Kaye, harassed by cancer, commencing her huge novel, which lies 400,000 unwritten words ahead of her, assuming as she does so that she will complete the task—or at all events that she has

---

4. It is, of course, also found in the white jazz culture, as in the virtuosity of jazz violinist Stephane Grappelli, at seventy-three, in concert with the equally exuberant classical master, Yehudi Menuhin, at sixty-seven.

no option: she must do it. She proceeds as though certain that she and the novel will survive to the end of it; that is, she lives in what Alfred North Whitehead has called "the sacred present." And she follows in a tradition symbolized by Robert Louis Stevenson who, himself wracked continuously by illness through his creative life, wrote in the closing passages of *Aes Triplex:* "By all means begin your folio" (quoted in McLeish 1976). Begin it, he meant, even if the actual completion for some reason is actually in doubt. Nor is ultimate public recognition necessary to the ultimate glory of the enterprise. In my circle of friends in Toronto is a woman who in her seventies has written a long novel that has never been published. Still, her creative act is beautiful in itself; and published or not, a novelist is still a novelist.

We are encountering here the guts and the tenacity of the creative individual, and nothing symbolizes more movingly this stamina, this courage, than the little cameo drawn for us by Hugh Kenner (1965) of the novelist Percy Wyndham Lewis, nearly blind at seventy-one, writing his third last major novel: "In silence, hour after hour, dropping each page as it was completed into a deep wooden tray on the floor at his side" (p. vii). Or Renoir still painting lovely pictures at a great age, even though he was so crippled by arthritis that a special machine had to be devised for him to move his arms and hands—yet still painting with joy.

Even across the discouragement of time this tenacity exists: Gutenberg patiently searched for the key to the riddle of the printing press, which he found unexpectedly, years later, while watching some wine presses at work. Likewise it took a friend of mine, a poet, two years among many other distracting activities to finish an exquisite sonnet. The tenacity of the black naive painter Clementine Hunter to wait across almost a lifetime for the chance at last to paint in oils is still another example.[5] It is the "Yes I can" of the creator.

---

5. Thus Hunter at ninety-five (February 1980) told an interviewer: "Evenings I had always the cooking and the kids. But I used to watch Miss Alberta Kinsey painting flowers up at the big house, and it looked like something I could maybe do ... I couldn't buy canvas, so I started [at sixty] stretching cloths, working on old shoe boxes, or anything that would take the paint."

A few years ago there appeared a British novel and film titled *The Loneliness of the Long Distance Runner*. The phrase has a poignant application also to many of us who are moving into and through our later years. Among the questions that I asked my thirty "private" creative adults was whether they were often lonely—a question dictated, no doubt, by my long-held conception that creativity is fed by loneliness. The answer from nearly all, which at first surprised me, is that they are rarely lonely. Then I realized that for the creative adult, although loneliness of course exists, even if only existential loneliness, it is loneliness in a new key. Creative people in their later years have had many experiences of loneliness, but they use loneliness rather than being used and abused by it. And they cherish the many opportunities of being alone, even though, again to my surprise, few of my private respondents reported that they worked in specified daily hours, what the French beautifully call "les heures sacrées."

I also sought from this private group whether they felt that among the hazards of later-life creativity were these: not enough time, not enough energy, not enough will power, and not enough encouragement. Among the respondents, neither lack of will nor lack of encouragement were cited as significant. A substantial group felt that lack of energy constituted a problem; and surprisingly enough, slightly more than half felt that lack of time was a problem in their creative lives.

As I reflect on this, I see that three influences are at work in this perceived lack of time. First, few older adults, even the more creative ones, are aware that for any given period of fifteen years after age sixty, assuming that ten hours a day are available for creative work of whatever kind, there are no fewer than 55,000 hours available. No one thinks about this. Second, creative people are also incorrigible planners, and often devoted fantasizers—and for some fantasies, no time is enough. Third, many nonprofessional creative adults are also giving out large sections of their time to other life activities: learning adventures, travel, passionate causes, social relations, and so on. No wonder they feel crowded for time in the special creative arena of their lives, and of course they may put some creativity into those other activities.

In fact, the conventional reasons for taking on new creative activities in the later years—removal of job responsibilities for men, loss of compelling family responsibilities for women—are echoed again and again in the responses from the private creators. Society, or social custom, suddenly gives permission to relinquish job and family commitments that especially to the generation over age sixty were sanctified almost as religious codes. For this enormous group of older adults, custom might have held them in channels of mandated routines until death, were it not that, especially in the case of men, they were compulsorily retired. Perhaps my colleague Foster Vernon has a point when he remarks occasionally that required retirement may be a blessing in disguise, for those who fear to let go to a new life.

It seems to be true that for many men and women a double permission is needed to enter the most fertile fields of their creative life. The second permission is their own: to give themselves permission, turning off at last the endlessly heard voices of the board of directors that is built into all our self-systems. To be freed by external circumstances from constraints of time and energy that have inhibited much of our unique creative life is not enough. We also need the inner freedom to choose unexpected creative fields, or within conventional creative arenas to perform with high individuality, with bravura and a certain braggart splendor. Since all creative adventures are good in later adulthood, to each must be his or her own. However, it is a pity if older adults, released at last for new creative exploits, settle for bland, timid, imitative actions and dry out their spirits in tired, unproductive routines when they might at last explore their own highly personal and deeply interesting and stimulating creativities.

This brings me to an issue that I find very challenging and very moving. It concerns in large measure those dear hearts whose frequent expression in the later years is, "I always meant to . . . ," who hover uncertainly in the border country of the creative life, not confident of their powers, confused by the myths, secretly mourning what they believe to be creative chances irretrievably lost, yet secretly still willing to enter the kingdom if it is possible. On various terms it is indeed possible, and in closing I want to suggest a few ways that this entrance might be realized.

Perhaps I should present a fantasy suggestion first, remarking as I do so that if it could ever be actualized it might also benefit many of us who feel ourselves to be well launched into later life creativity. The humanistic psychotherapist Sidney M. Jourard once wrote about the advantages of what he called "check-out places" for men and women in their middle and later years. These would be organized way stations on the life journey where adults feeling temporarily at the end of their tether, or feeling metaphorically or actually in disgrace with fortune and men's eyes, or desperately fatigued and unable to make out which of the next forks on the trail they should take, could find both physical and emotional healing and enlightenment for new lives and careers. Jourard does not specifically mention self-discovery and renewal through fresh insights into one's latent creative powers, but this is my present suggestion. It would be invaluable if there were checkout places that enabled adults at whatever age to assess their greater creative potentialities. It is a dream, but one must never underestimate the fallout from dreams. Besides, as with all fantasies, even in scaling it down into more manageable projects, we could gain much ground.

My second suggestion is quite practical and has some relationship to the first. I am astonished at the paucity of facilities available to adults on our continent who wish to study the whole creative process in some depth, and thereby help release their own special talents more effectively. I am not referring here to instamatic courses on how to sell better, though there is nothing wrong with helping salespeople improve their sales. I am referring instead to the type of experience offered by the School of Continuing Studies at my own university and at all too few other centers, which considers simultaneously selfhood and the creative process, and which moves from the theory of creativity to the joy and release of many creative games. In later adulthood we need to use the values of games for vitalizing mind and body and advancing fantasy and creativity. (If we need an example of a game that, except for promoting sociability, is wholly unproductive, I think I would nominate Bingo. I lament the case of those men and women who may find themselves trapped in an eternal Bingo scene. Part of their creative adventure is to escape the trap.)

I have another cause that is neither won nor lost—a creative life strategy that can do much to preserve the juices of the creative life; and this is the regular keeping of a personal reflective journal. When I urge the values of journal keeping in my own seminars of about thirty people, perhaps four or five will take up the idea and make it part of their life. Still, I am not discouraged. By a personal reflective journal I mean much more than a diary of events, though that is valuable, since otherwise our days melt behind us into a blurred stream like the unreproducible months of hundreds of television and radio programs seen and heard and forgotten, and things worth remembering, but forgotten, from the press.

Successful journal keeping, the kind that vitalizes us and helps keep flowing the springs of our creative instincts, involves keeping in a small hardcover notebook a daily record of ideas one wants to remember, creative ideas otherwise lost in the maze of the unconscious: unusual little incidents, small cameos of people, snatches of beauty from the environment, flights of birds, some unexpected glimpses of nature and human nature, absurd moments and thoughts, words read that one wants to recall, and reflections, usually compassionate and wise with the accumulating wisdom of the years, on the actions and thoughts of one's self. One need not be a literary person to keep such a journal. However, to keeping my own journal I attribute the ease with which after many years of not writing fiction, I was able to resume with a 12,000-word novella during the past spring.

Finally, those of us who are already seekers need to assume and maintain the role of believers in our own creativity, whatever it may be; and also the role of encouragers of others. We need to serve as role models for many who even in our private environments are silently observing us and finding stimulus and courage to take creative steps because we are maintaining our creativity in projects, human relationships, and learning. And we also in turn require role models—men and women whose lives and words reinvigorate us when, as always happens, we encounter temporary periods of flatness and discouragement.

The sublime topic we have been reviewing brings together the Ulyssean concept, the joy of lifelong learning, and the good news of the lifelong potential of creative powers. Therefore I close with three illustrative concepts.

The first is the creed of the Ulyssean Society, which is printed on each membership card and reads as follows:

> As a Companion of The Ulyssean Society, I am committed to the noble concept and the provable fact that men and women in the middle and later years can, if they choose to do so, richly maintain the powers to produce, to learn, and to create, until the very end of the life journey.

The second is a quotation from the great modern French writer André Gide who in his last week at age eighty-four in 1947 was busily engaged in improving his Latin and in maintaining his wonderful journal: "It is a rule of life that when one door closes, another always opens. But most of us spend so much time mourning the losses behind the closed doors that we seldom see—let alone grasp—the opportunities presented by the newly opened doors."

And the third is a remark by the American painter James Chapin, who in his late life developed a love affair for Toronto and died there in 1973, still painting fine large canvases at age eighty-eight. Chapin said to a circle of young artists who surrounded him, enchanted by his age and creativity: "Be careful that you prepare well for the years from sixty to eighty-plus. You will find that they can be the best years of your life."

REFERENCES

Adler, Alfred. 1965. *Superiority and Social Interest*. London: Routledge and Kegan Paul.

Arieti, Silvano. 1976. *Creativity: The Magic Synthesis*. New York: Holt, Reinhart & Winston.

Barron, Frank. 1963. *Creativity and Psychological Health*. New York: Van Nostrand.

Burnshaw, Stanley. 1970. *The Seamless Web*. New York: Braziller.

Butcher, H.J. 1968. *Human Intelligence: Its Nature and Assessment*. London: Methuen.

De Bono, Edward. 1967. *The Use of Lateral Thinking*. London: Jonathan Cape.

Donahue, Wilma, and C. Tibbitts. 1957. *The New Frontiers of Aging*. Ann Arbor: University of Michigan Press.

Douglas, A. Vibert. 1956. *The Life of Arthur Stanley Eddington*. London: Nelson.

Fromm, E. 1959. "The Creative Attitude." In *Creativity and Its Cultivation*, edited by H.H. Anderson. New York: Harper & Row.

Gardner, John W. 1964. *Self-Renewal: The Individual and the Innovative*. New York: Harper & Row.

Getzel, J.W., and P.W. Jackson. 1962. *Creativity and Intelligence*. New York: Wiley.

Gross, Ronald, 1977. *The Lifelong Learner*. New York: Simon and Schuster.

Haefele, J.W. 1962. *Creativity and Innovation*. New York: Holt, Reinhart & Winston.

Horney, Karen. 1950. *Neurosis and Human Growth*. New York: Norton.

Houle, Cyril. 1961. *The Inquiring Mind*. Madison: University of Wisconsin Press.

Kenner, Hugh. 1965. "Introduction" to *Self-Condemned*. Chicago: Henry Regnery.

Koestler, Arthur. 1969. *The Ghost in the Machine*. London: Hutchinson.

Kubie, L.S. 1958. *Neurotic Distortion of the Creative Process*. Lawrence: University of Kansas Press.

Maslow, Abraham. 1959. "Creativity in Self-Actualizing People." In *Creativity and Its Cultivation*, edited by H.H. Anderson. New York: Harper & Row.

McLeish, John A.B. 1976. *The Ulyssean Adult*. New York: McGraw-Hill.

Restak, Richard. 1979. *The Brain: The Last Frontier*. New York: Doubleday.

Roe, Anne. 1952. *The Making of a Scientist*. New York: Dodd, Mead.

Rogers, C. 1959. "Toward a Theory of Creativity." In *Creativity and Its Cultivation*, edited by H.H. Anderson, pp. 000–00. New York: Harper & Row.

Taylor, Calvin W. and J. Holland. 1964. "Predicators of Creative Performance." In *Creativity: Progress and Potential*, edited by Calvin W. Taylor. New York: McGraw-Hill.

Torrance, E. Paul. 1963. *Education and the Creative Potential*. Minneapolis: University of Minnesota Press.

Tuska, C.K. 1955. "Increasing Inventive Creativeness." *Journal of the Franklin Institute* 260:93–98.

6 A LITERARY PERSPECTIVE

May Sarton

At first the subject of creativity and aging troubled me. I found that I did not want to write about that. I wanted to read poems, my own poems, celebrating old age. But I finally admonished myself: "Sarton, you are not getting at this task. You are not doing what you are supposed to do." And what I was supposed to do—or so I imagined—was to write about the sweetness of creativity as one grows older, and how much easier it gets. Does it? I turned to a page in *Journal of a Solitude* where I had quoted these words by Humphrey Trevelyan on Goethe:

> It seems that two qualities are necessary if a great artist is to remain creative to the end of a long life; he must on the one hand retain an abnormally keen awareness of life, he must never grow complacent, never be content with life, must always demand the impossible and when he cannot have it, must despair. The burden of the mystery must be with him day and night. He must be shaken by the naked truths that will not be comforted. This divine discontent, this disequilibrium, this state of inner tension is the source of artistic energy. Many lesser poets have it only in their youth; some even of the greatest lose it in middle life. Wordsworth lost the courage to despair and with it his poetic power. [And you remember how very dull his later poems are.] But more often the

117

dynamic tensions are so powerful that they destroy the man before he reaches maturity.

It is not surprising, then, that six of the poets of my time have committed suicide. The poet's life is not often a merry one. So I cannot write about a pleasant kind of wisdom that descends like a mantle after sixty, but rather of a continuing attempt to deal with conflict, and unfortunately, conflict does not go away. It is always there and from it may spring the psychic energy which drives one to create. One of the conflicts that does not go away is that between art and life. How am I to make the time to do my work when I have to answer fifty letters a week? But if conflict is inevitable, the joy of creation itself never dies. Let us place this beside Trevelyan's account of the creative person.

Birthday Present

Renewal cannot be picked
Like a daffodil
In a swift gesture,
Cannot be cut like a pussy willow
And brought into the house.
It cannot even be imagined
Like the blue sky
We have not seen for days.

But we can be helped toward it.
True love gave me time,
Gave me, for myself alone,
This whole open day
We would have spent together.

True love gave me this—
Harder to find
Than a hummingbird's nest,
Rare as the elusive
Scent of arbutus
Under sodden leaves,
More welcome than a cup

Of spring water
After long drought.

I hold it in my hands,
I breathe it in,
I drink it,
While fifty-nine years
Of ardor and tenderness,
Of struggle and creation—
The whole complex bundle—
Falls away in a streak of light
Like a shooting star,
As the soul,
Unencumbered,
Alive, ageless,
Meets the pristine moment:
Poetry again.

The pristine moment does not happen every day, but when it comes it is timeless. That is the marvelous, ageless joy of creation.

It's much in my mind these days that many of my contemporaries and friends are swamped by having to maintain a big house or garden for which they no longer have the strength. But a work of art is created once and for all, and does not have to be maintained. It takes place outside of time, it will never age, and while one is writing a poem or painting a painting, one is living in the eternal present like a saint. One forgets arthritis or rheumatism or the lines on one's face. It doesn't matter that the pace is slow if the work is going to be good. One is tapping a source that runs very deep and is outside time. And of course this is immensely joyful. I am never as happy and absorbed as when I am struggling to get a poem down. "Why do you get into a poem?" Robert Frost was asked, and he answered: "In order to get out!" The "getting out" is the fun.

It occurs to me that it may be easier for artists to grow old than for professional people who, at retirement, are often forcibly cut off from the routines that sustain and give meaning to life, cut off just when they have a great deal to give, more perhaps than ever before in their lives. But old artists do not fade away, they ripen. The personality has been developing along the same line for many years and nothing of it has to be restricted or given up because of age.

I feel a holy joy when I evoke Matisse in his eighties, lying in bed, his arthritic hands tied to long brushes, making those magnificent geometric designs that we see now in the museum in Washington and elsewhere. Georgia O'Keefe at ninety is still productive and feisty. Verdi wrote Falstaff when he was eighty. W. B. Yeats achieved some of his greatest poems and developed a new style when he was an old man. There is also Thomas Hardy who decided that he was going to write only poems—and here I feel for him—because the reviews of his novels had been so devastating. He wrote great poems when he was an old man.

What makes it possible for creativity to stay alive when the body is already disintegrating, when the physical self is becoming a burden? For one thing, as I've suggested, it's easy to go on doing what one has always done. I've observed this with gardeners. Basil DeSelincourt, the literary critic, was a great gardener, and he went on being able to put in a vegetable garden, doing the whole thing, when he was in his late eighties, because he'd always done it and the muscles were there. If you've always drawn or you've always written poems, you are deeply grooved in that direction.

But perhaps the signature of the artist is first of all an exceptional psychic energy. My mother suffered from many psychosomatic illnesses, ailments such as tachycardia, migraine headaches, terrible, waking almost every morning with a sick headache, and at the end of her life, got cancer from which she died. But she had inside her a flame of psychic energy that never dimmed or failed and she went on creating till the very end. The technical term for this, I suppose, is motivation. Any artist is highly motivated. He is driven to do what he does. He did not choose to be a poet, he was chosen to be one. So while physical energy may diminish, psychic energy is far more durable. The soul does remain ageless, thank God.

What all this amounts to is that the artist or writer has the tools, the craft, in his grasp. And as long as the psychic energy is there, the drive to create remains fresh and alive and he's going to go on willy-nilly. This is really why I found the subject hard to confront because it seemed to me either you do or you don't. You either have this psychic energy and have always had it, or you don't have it and then you'll never have it. It is not just an easy pattern that you can develop later on. It has to be there from the beginning to some extent.

But perhaps the greatest problem—there has to be a problem after all, since we are on earth, not in heaven—is that if one is a creator and has gone on producing for forty years as I have, there is a certain amount of pure business stuff that has to be faced and responded to every day. The clutter is the problem. The more famous you are, the more clamorous all these demands and requests that come from the outside at a time when you no longer have unlimited energy. Increasing responsibility toward the public can silt up the clear waters of creation.

Of course it's here that aging demands that we become less compulsive, that we learn to accept limitations and not feel guilt about them. The creator must remain to some degree passionate in his desire to create, even as he tries to become more detached. It's a fascinating adventure, is it not?—the conflict between art and life that is never solved. Every single day when I go to my desk, if I am working on a book, I engage in a battle with myself. There is that woman who is sitting beside her dying mother's bed who wrote to me yesterday and said, "What am I going to do about the silence afterwards?" And I say to myself, "Sarton, you have to answer that letter." But another Sarton says, "Yes, Sarton, but you have to write your book." And there is again the excruciating conflict. I see no solution, alas, except to try to do them both.

I'm not an expert, and that's why it's so hard for me to write about all this in generalities. I am close to old age, although I'm teased by my friends in their eighties for daring to call sixty-eight old! It is the infancy of old age, they tell me. Very well, some things *are* easier. I've written thirty-five books and lost some of the acute anguish of my youth, when I felt guilty about not doing something truly useful, such as teaching deprived children or going into politics. That conflict about whether I can justify the time to write my books, instead of doing something useful, has been softened by the knowledge

that in a different way the work has been useful. And the letters that I complain about so much have also released that
burden of anxiety about the worth of what I'm doing. But no
writer or artist, no true one, ever believes wholly in his talent.
Every new book is a new challenge, a possible disaster, and
everything that he has done before is to some extent the enemy of what he is doing now.

It is balm for me as I get older to see my work touch and
give courage to the young. And this drives me to want to do
better, to open more doors, to try at least to exemplify what an
ongoing life can be and can mean even into old age. And what
makes it ongoing is, of course, the necessity to keep on examining experience by means of the creation of a work of art. In
my journals I often quote Florida Scott Maxwell, especially
that marvelous book, *The Measure of My Days*. Before I pro-
ceed to poems, I must quote one passage from her that I found
the other day:

> If I suffer from my lacks, and I do daily, I also feel elation at what
> I have become. At times I feel a sort of intoxication because of
> some small degree of gain, as though the life that is in me has
> been my charge, the trust birth brought me. And my blunders,
> sins, the blanks in me as well as the gifts have in some long pain-
> ful transmutation made the life that is in me clearer.

And that's what it's all about, isn't it? It is what we are all
trying to do, to clarify, to get down deeper, to be more honest
with ourselves and so to make the life in us clearer.

I have always looked forward to old age, and the reason, as
the poems make clear, is that I have known so many great
old people. Well, I looked forward to old age wrongly because
I imagined it would be serene and uncluttered, and rightly
because it would make it possible for me to grow and to create poems and books that have growth in them. I am convinced that we are on earth to make our souls. And to that
extent old age, of course, is the most thrilling time of all. Because we are coming close to an end, this conviction that the
making of the soul is of paramount importance is very much
with us. As a young woman, I was lucky to know and love so
many distinguished, fruitful, creative old people, some of
them not creative in the ordinary sense of producing books or

works of art, but creative as livers of life. And so I want to
end this essay with a celebration of the old, as I have known
them. I'll begin with a quotation from W. B. Yeats: "Think
where man's glory most begins and ends./And say my glory
was I had such friends."

The first poem is *The Great Transparencies*. This is not
about an individual person, it is about many. It happens in old
age, I think, that one becomes more transparent because one is
less self-conscious, because one is able to admit vulnerability
and becomes less defensive.

The Great Transparencies

Lately I have been thinking much of those,
The open ones, the great transparencies,
Through whom life—is it wind or water?—
    flows
Unstinted, who have learned the sovereign
    ease.
They are not young; they are not ever young.

Youth is too vulnerable to bear the tide,
And let it rise, and never hold it back,
Then let it ebb, not suffering from pride,
Nor thinking it must ebb from private lack.
The elders yield because they are so strong—

Seized by the great wind like a ripening field,
All rippled over in a sensuous sweep,
Wave after wave, lifted and glad to yield,
But whether wind or water, never keep
The tide from flowing or hold it back for long.

Lately I have been thinking much of these,
The unafraid although still vulnerable,
Through whom life flows, the great
    transparencies,
The old and open, brave and beautiful . . .
They are not young; they are not ever young.

I shall celebrate next an Indian friend of mine with whom I could not communicate in words because we did not speak the same language, an Indian of the Pueblos in Santa Fe who worked for a dear friend of mine, Edith Warner. His name was Tilano. He worked for her, and brought in the wood, and did odd jobs. But they were truly friends and when he became very old, she brought him into the house—he had lived in his pueblo before—and opened up a big window in the adobe wall so that he could watch the sun set.

Letter to an Indian Friend

Was it a long journey for you to begin
To grow peaceful green things,
To harvest well, to watch the sun
Go down, to find the ancient springs?
What human pain, what wild desire
Did you burn in the fire,
Long ago, Tilano?

What is the first step, Tilano,
Toward the wisdom of your feet,
Treading the dust or the snow
So quiet, so tender, so fleet?
I have come from far
To the warm sun and the shelter,
A long journey to reach here,
And now it is clear
That I do not know
The first step.

What is the first act, Tilano,
Toward the wisdom of your hands?
They plant the corn;
They bring in the lamp in the evening,
Wood for the fire, and each thing done
With rigorous love, with devotion.
It was a long journey to you and the sun,
And now it seems I clasp in your hand
A land of work and silence, a whole land.

What is the first prayer, Tilano?
To go into the forest
And be content to sit
For many days alone,
Not asking God to come,
Since He is present in the sun,
Simple and quiet in the tree and stone,
How many times have you watched the sun
    rise
That when I look into your eyes,
So old, so old and gay, I see there
That I have never learned the first prayer?

Then there was Koteliansky. S.S. Koteliansky was the great friend of Katherine Mansfield, of D.H. Lawrence; he adored Katherine Mansfield. He was like a prophet from the Old Testament, a fierce pure Jew with fire in his eyes who was absolutely incorruptible. And the letters that Katherine Mansfield wrote Kot always were on a rather different level from those that she wrote to other people; some of the affectation and self-consciousness were not there. You could not do that with Kot, you had to be very honest. He was poor when I knew him, living in St. John's Wood in London. And I went always for tea and there he would be, sitting smoking his Russian cigarettes in the kitchen, back to the tiny stove, tea carefully laid out, Russian tea in glasses. Sometimes James Stephens joined us and then we drank gin with buffalo grass in it in the Russian way. Stephens would get drunk and so would I, while he recited poetry for hours. But the best times, though I was fond of James Stephens, were when I saw Kot alone. And the best of all was thinking about him in his house, surrounded by the things he loved, and being most himself.

Kot's House

If the house is clean and pure,
Fiercely incorruptible
God is ever at the door,
The Father and the Prodigal.
Should He never be aware

Of the order of each plate,
Still they will be shining there
And the floor immaculate.

Though at times the things revolt,
Fickle water or damp wall,
The chipped cup or stiffened bolt
(Love, where is your Prodigal?)

Still the house waits and is glad;
Every tea cup is welcome,
Every cup aspires to God
Even if He never come.

And whether He exist at all,
The Father and the Prodigal,
He is expected by these things
And each plate Hosannah sings!

It brings Kot back so to me! Of course I did terrible things. When you're old, you learn some things that when you're young, you really can't know yet. Although I had appreciated the immaculateness of Kot's house, I stayed there once when I couldn't find a hotel and I spilled some powder when I was powdering my nose. I had slept in the dining room, on a cot. The spilled powder horrified Kot and you would have thought that it was the Augean stable at least! One is careless sometimes when one is young.

Then, of course there was my mother, from whom I learned so much and about so many different things that it's hard even to begin to talk about them, and it's been hard to write about her. But in the case of this poem, I found the image. Not saying my mother was wonderful because of this and that, but just seeing her in the garden.

An Observation

True gardeners cannot bear a glove
Between the sure touch and the tender root,

Must let their hands grow knotted as they
    move
With a rough sensitivity about
Under the earth, between the rock and shoot,
Never to bruise or wound the hidden fruit.
And so I watched my mother's hands grow
    scarred,
She who could heal the wounded plant or
    friend
With the same vulnerable yet rigorous love;
I minded once to see her beauty gnarled,
But now her truth is given to me to live,
As I learn for myself we must be hard
To move among the tender with an open
    hand,
And to stay sensitive up to the end
Pay with some toughness for a gentle world.

Now to a very different woman from my mother. She is
Camille Mayran, whom I've been corresponding with for thirty
or forty years. She's now in her nineties. She was a very famous writer in France before World War II, and won the Prix
Femina-Vie-Heureuse. But when I knew her she had been
through two world wars, twice seen her house totally de-
stroyed, her husband dead of tuberculosis as a result of World
War I, all her books, everything gone. When I knew her, she
was living a life of great beauty on a small farm in the South
of France with very, very little materially.

Joy in Provence

For Camille Mayran

I found her, rich loser of all,
Whom two wars have stripped to the bone,
High up on her terrace wall
Over vineyards asleep in the sun—
Her riches, the ample scene
Composed in the barn's round door;
Her riches, rough cliff and pine,

Aromatic air—and no more.
Here, seasoned and sweetened by loss,
She thrives like thyme in the grass.

This woman's feet are so light,
So light the weight of her eyes
When she walks her battlements late
To harvest her thoughts as they rise,
She is never caught, only wise.
She rests on the round earth's turning
And follows the radiant skies,
Then reads Pascal in the morning.
And, walking beside her, I learned
How those dazzling silences burned.

On the longest day of June,
When summer wanes as it flowers
And dusk folds itself into dawn,
We had shared the light drenched hours.
We lay on rough rock in the sun,
Conversing till words were rare,
Conversing till words were done,
High up in the pungent air,
Then silently paced while the moon
Rose to dance her slow pavane.

The wine from a meditation
Was mine to drink deeply that night,
O vintage severe, and elation
To be pressed out of loss, and from light!
Alive to her thought, yet alone,
As I lay in my bed, close to prayer,
A whisper came and was gone:
"Rejoice" and the word in the air.
But when the silence was broken,
Not by me, not by her, who had spoken?

Now I come to a complete contrast. She was an extremely beautiful woman, a raving beauty, who should have been a great actress. I base Sybil, the character in *A Reckoning*, more

or less on this woman, whose name was Rosalind Greene. I
was enormously susceptible to her beauty when I was a child.
(The Greenes were one of the families I adopted. I was always
adopting families because I was an only child myself.) When
she was seventy-five they gave a party for her and I wrote this
poem. Everybody was so terrified that I would read it and that
it might not work, that it was excruciating. Her son-in-law
kept saying, "Do you really think you should read it?" He was
a very tall man looking down at me, and I kept saying, "But I
want to read it, I wrote it for this day." Well, I read it, of
course, and Rosalind sat there, at seventy-five still so beautiful, with tears streaming down her cheeks.

For Rosalind on her Seventy-Fifth Birthday

Tonight we come to praise
Her splendor, not her years,
Pure form and what it burns—
Who teaches this or learns?—
Intrinsic, beyond tears,
Splendor that has no age.
Take your new-fangled beauties off the stage!

The high point of the throat
That dazzled every heart—
Who was not young and awed
By beauty so unflawed

It seemed not life, but art?—
Terrible as a swan
Young children, deeply moved, might look
    upon.

The blazing sapphire eyes—
They looked out from a queen.
Yet there was wildness near;
She glimmered like a deer
No hunter could bring down.
So warm, so wild, so proud

      She moved among us like a light-brimmed
         cloud.

      The way her dresses flowed!
      So once in Greece, so once . . .
      Passion and its control.
      She drew many a soul
      To join her in the dance.
      Give homage fierce as rage.
      Take your new-fangled beauties off the stage!

   We talk about old people in a sort of lump. You know,
"What are we to do with the old people?" That's one reason I
wanted to collect a whole set of old marvelous people as different from each other as they can be. You can't really do anything about anybody in a lump—blacks in a lump, old people
in a lump, Chicanos in a lump.
   Here is a rather different kind of poem, a letter to Marynia
Farnham, with whom I had some therapy a few years ago. She
was then retired, over seventy, and still very great as a
therapist.

         Christmas Letter to a Psychiatrist, 1970

                     1

      These bulbs forgotten in a cellar,
      Pushing up through the dark their wan white
         shoots,
      Trying to live—their hopeless hope
      Has been with me like an illness
      The image of what tries to be born
      For twenty years or more,
      But dies for lack of light.

      Today I saw it again in the stare
      Of the homeless cat, that hunger
      Not for food only, but to be taken in,
      And to trust enough to risk it . . .
      Shelter, life itself. Can I tame her?
      Come the worst cold, will she freeze?

How marvelous to know you can save,
Restore, nourish the abandoned,
That the life line is there
In your wise hands, Marynia!

2

"Yes," you say, "of course at Christmas
Half the world is suicidal."
And you are there. You answer the phone—
The wry voice with laughter in it.
Again and again the life line is thrown out.
There is no end to the work of salvage
In the drowning high seas of Christmas
When loneliness, in the name of Christ
(That longing!), attacks the world.

3

One by one, they come from their wilderness
Like shy wild animals
Weeping blood from their wounds,
Wounds they dare not look at
And cannot bind or heal alone.
What is it that happens then
In the small room
Where someone listens,
Where someone answers,
Where someone cares,
Whom they cannot hurt
With their sharp infant teeth,
With their sharp old antlers?

What does she do,
This doctor, this angel,
Who holds so many
In her human hands?
How does she heal the animal pain
So the soul may live?

4

No Ceres, she, no Aphrodite;
She cannot provide the harvest
Nor the longed-for love.

This angel must be anarchic,
Fierce, full of laughter,
Will neither punish
Nor give absolution,
Is always acute, sometimes harsh.
Still the impersonal wing
Does shelter, provides a place, a climate
Where the soul can meet itself at last.

There is no way out,
Only the way deeper and deeper inward.
There are no solutions,
But every word is action,
As is every silence.
On a good day the patient
Has used his reason
To cut through secret evasions,
Secret fears,
Has experienced himself
As a complex whole.

But angels do not operate
By any means we can define.
They come when they are needed.
(I can tell you of the resonance,
The beat of wings
Threshing out truth
Long after the hour is past.)
When they have gone
The light-riddled spirit
Is as alone as ever,
But able to fly its course again
Through the most hostile sky.

5

I know what it is like, Marynia.
Once I watched a jay flopping, helpless,
In the snow outside this window—
I brought it in, managed to pull out the quill
Shot through just under the eye.
I know what it is to have to be brutal
Toward the badly crippled
In order to set them free.
Then it was Easter and I saw the jay
Fly off whole into the resurrected air.

Now it is Christmas
When infant love, vulnerable beyond our
        knowing,
Is born again to save the world.

And for whatever crucifixions it will suffer.
Angel, be blessed for your wings.

Marynia died the other day, I saw in the *New York Times*.
    Well, much longer ago than that, when I was very young
and still in the theater, I had a friend called Lugné-Poë, a
great theater director in Paris who brought Ibsen to Paris in
the 1890s and who was a tower of strength for artists and theater people all over the world. Lugné would start his day by
sending cables to perhaps ten people, including me sometimes,
saying, "Now don't give up. We need you, Sarton." One tele-
gram would go to the Argentine, one would go to Germany,
and so on. Marvelous. Lugné-Poë died just before the Germans
took France in 1940. Thank goodness he died before it happened, but he had foreseen that everything was going to
pieces, that the morale was low. I was struggling then to keep
a small theater company together and when these words, often
called, reached me out of the blue when things looked so bad,
it lifted me up. I think about him a great deal in other contexts. It is long, long ago since I had anything to do with theater, and now, of course, I am almost as old as he was when he
died. But he still gives me courage.

What the Old Man Said

At sixty-five said, "I fight every day.
My dear, nothing but death will stop
My uninterrupted élan in the play."
Than wrote, "When I am forced to see
What happens to our old humanity,
All seems ignoble and I rage
To have been listed player on this stage."
At sixty-five that anger conquered fear:
The old man raged, but he did not despair.

At sixty-seven then he laughed and said,
"My dear, how proud I am of all the haters
Who stand behind and wish that I were
      dead,"
Those who had tasted of his honesty,
Those usurers of mediocrity—
At sixty-seven he refused to praise
(And lost his job) their rotten little plays.
But when he told me how he shouted there,
The old man laughed, but he did not despair.

At seventy said, "We must work, my dear.
I see a certain look upon their faces.
Discouragement? Perhaps I dream it there.
The wicked times have put me back to school,
And I shall die a sensitive young fool.
The news is doing me to death at last."

And then a note, "The evil eats me fast.
You must help men not to be slaves, my
      dear!"
(The old man died, but he did not despair.)

I've gone back to that many times.
   I wanted to end with a couple of poems about where I am
now. Here is one called *A Recognition for Perley Cole*. Some
good poems begin in anger. No poem, perhaps, ends in anger
because poetry is a little bit like prayer, I think: you may be-

gin a prayer in anger, but it doesn't end there. And I was very angry about a bad review, and that gave me the steam to write the poem, I guess. Perley Cole was the farmer who worked for me in Nelson. Here again we come to the magic of images. I put together with Perley, a New England farmer, Brancusi, a sculptor whom I had known in Paris. You remember how sophisticated his work is, the famous *Flight,* these metallic shining things that he created which are in all the museums. He was a peasant, Brancusi was, a Romanian peasant who walked to Paris, made his way, lived on nothing, and so it seemed sort of a nice putting together of Perley Cole and Brancusi, who was an old man when I knew him, too.

A Recognition

I wouldn't know how rare they come these
    days,
But I know Perley's rare. I know enough
To stop fooling around with words, and praise
This man who swings a scythe in subtle ways,
And brings green order, carved out of the
    rough.
I wouldn't know how rare, but I discover
They used to tell an awkward learning boy,
"Keep the heel down, son, careful of the
    swing!"

I guess at perils and peril makes me sing.
So let the world go, but hold fast to joy,
And praise the craftsman till Hell freezes
    over!
I watched him that first morning when the
    dew
Still slightly bent tall, toughened grasses,
Sat up in bed to watch him coming through
Holding the scythe so lightly and so true
In slow sweeps and in lovely passes,
The swing far out, far out—but not too far,
The pause to wipe and whet the shining
    blade.

I felt affinities: farmer and poet
Share a good deal, although they may not
    know it.
It looked as easy as when the world was
    made,
And God could pull a bird out or a star.

For there was Perley in his own sweet way
Pulling some order out of ragged land,
Cutting the tough, chaotic growth away,
So peace could saunter down a summer day,
For here comes Cole with genius in his hand!
I saw in him a likeness to that flame,
Brancusi, in his Paris studio,
Who pruned down, lifted from chaotic night
Those naked, shining images of flight—
The old man's gentle malice and bravado,
Boasting hard times: "It was my game!"

"*C'était mon jeu!*"—to wrest joy out of pain,
The endless skillful struggle to uncloud
The clouded vision, to reduce and prune,
And bring back from the furnace, fired again,
A world of magic, joy alone allowed.
Now Perley says, "God damn it!"—and much
    worse.
Hearing him, I get back some reverence.
Could you, they ask, call such a man your
    friend?
Yes (damn it!), and yes world without end!
Brancusi's game and his make the same
    sense,
And not unlike a prayer is Perley's curse.

So let the rest go, and heel down, my boy,
And praise the artist till Hell freezes over,
For he is rare, he with his scythe (no toy),
He with his perils, with his skill and joy,
Who comes to prune, to make clear, to
    uncover,

The old man, full of wisdom, in his prime.
There in the field, watching him as he passes,
I recognize that violent, gentle blood,
Impatient patience. I would, if I could,
Call him my kin, there scything down the
     grasses,
Call him my good luck in a dirty time.

And a last poem, to round it off:

On a Winter Night

On a winter night
I sat alone
In a cold room,
Feeling old, strange
At the year's change,
In fire light.

Last fire of youth,
All brilliance burning,
And my year turning—
One dazzling rush,
Like a wild wish
Or blaze of truth.

First fire of age,
And the soft snow
Of ash below—
For the clean wood
The end was good;
For me, an image.

For then I saw
That fires, not I,
Burn down and die;
That flare of gold
Turns old, turns cold.
Not I. I grow.

Nor old, nor young,
The burning sprite
Of my delight,
A salamander
In fires of wonder,
Gives tongue, gives tongue!

7 SOME THOUGHTS FROM A FOLK CULTURAL PERSPECTIVE

Alan Jabbour

It occurred to me recently that within a mile or two of my childhood home in Jacksonville, Florida, stood a handsome building with the name "Old Folks Home" proudly emblazoned in large letters across the portico. For all I know the building and the name still stand, but as I think now of the name "Old Folks Home," it has an oddly old-fashioned ring to my ears. The last twenty years have certainly been turbulent terminologically where old people are concerned, and our uncertainty about what to call old people doubtless reflects our deeper uncertainty about their place in our society. You can imagine, then, with what hesitation I approach addressing the subject under the auspices of an institute devoted to the study of aging. Not only am I likely to use the wrong terms, but I represent a federal institution, the American Folklife Center, and a professional network, folklorists, both of which contain embedded in them that odd and old-fashioned word "folk." To overcome this vague discomfort, I shall do what we folklorists study: I'll tell some stories, hoping through them to share some thoughts on the subject in order to begin bridging the gap between students of folklore and students of aging.

We may begin by framing the storytelling with three questions:

1. Can folk arts serve as a touchstone to unlock creativity in old people?
2. If they can, what benefits are there to old people in encouraging folk arts (or more broadly, *folklife*) among them?
3. What benefits are there for society at large?

To these overarching questions, let me append the definition of "folklife" included in the authorizing legislation of the American Folklife Center, so that my personal and institutional point of view will be clearer:

> The term "American folklife" means the traditional expressive culture shared within the various groups in the United States: familial, ethnic, occupational, religious, regional; expressive culture includes a wide range of creative and symbolic forms such as custom, belief, technical skill, language, literature, art, architecture, music, play, dance, drama, ritual, pageantry, handicraft; these expressions are mainly learned orally, by imitation, or in performance, and are generally maintained without benefit of formal instruction or institutional direction.

TAPPING CREATIVE WELLSPRINGS IN THE ELDERLY

Folklorist Gladys-Marie Fry, whose study *Nightriders in Black Folk History* (1975) explicates the tradition and significance of stories about "night doctors" in Southern Afro-American folklore, told me recently that she had had two extraordinary experiences while interviewing elderly black folks on the subject. Twice she was visiting rest homes for the elderly in the Washington, D.C., area, in order to interview them for stories about the "night doctors" who kidnapped or murdered people for medical experimentation. As she moved from one person to the next, she came upon an old woman who the nurses indicated was hopelessly senile, "out of it," perhaps crazy, and certainly unable to utter a coherent sentence. But on proceeding to state her subject, she discovered that the older patient indeed could and did talk, summoning up narrative accounts in halting but quite coherent sentences. She responded to the folklore subject Professor Fry raised, and she could parse her sentences. All this (stories being as they are) evoked great astonishment among the assembled doctors and nurses, who vowed the woman had not uttered an intelligible sentence in years.

What are we to make of this story? Is it yet another instance in the dreary litany of our inexcusable neglect of the aged? Had the old lady simply lapsed into incoherence as a result of neglect, contempt, and studied inattention, thus fulfilling in fact the role society had prescribed for her as a superfluous nonperson? Perhaps. But as a folklorist, I derive a somewhat different moral from the story. Please bear in mind that I put forth this example not as a scientist reporting conclusions, but as a storyteller evoking hunches. What the story means to me is that folklore and folk arts touch and speak to a deep-coursing stream in the human psyche. Or, to look at it the other way around, folklore *is* the deep-coursing stream in the psyche, and to evoke the folklore is to call forth the expression, the formal articulation, of that wellspring. When Professor Fry asked the question about nightriders, she was successful in eliciting a response, not simply because she was sympathetic, or showed warmth, interest, and human concern, but because she *said the magic word.*

I can add to the story a less dramatic anecdote from my own life. In the mid-1960s I had the transforming experience of studying the art of old-time fiddling with a splendid master fiddler, Henry Reed of Glen Lyn, Virginia. Mr. Reed, who has since died, was born, reared, and spent most of his life along the Virginia/West Virginia border. He was in his early eighties when I knew him, and was subject to a few of the infirmities of age. One was a sort of palsy, which a physician once labeled for me and pronounced correctable, but which was never corrected before his death. At family meals he managed his fork and spoon only with considerable effort (and occasional misfires). Drinking a mug of coffee required two hands to maneuver the mug, coffee sloshing within it, to his mouth. All this was viewed by him and the rest of the household with equanimity and good humor—old age had its vexations, he might have said, but he remained the active head of an active household, and life also provided abundant satisfactions.

The point I want to make is that though he could drink his coffee only with difficulty, he still played the fiddle elegantly.

There was a bit of scratch and surface noise, to be sure, partly because of the instrument itself, partly because he was rusty for lack of regular practice, but partly also because of the palsy and the general stiffness one associates with age. His friend Oscar Wright, ten years his junior and a fervent admirer of Henry Reed's playing for fifty years, would whisper to me, "You should have heard him thirty years ago." Nevertheless, his elaborate and complicated style of bowing and fingering the fiddle—a living testimony to the older musical art of the frontier Upper South—was essentially unaltered, uncompromised by the palsy. I would often watch him raise the bow, shaking visibly, to the fiddle, then listen in awe as the music, once begun, poured out with unhesitating agility and mellifluousness.

How did he do it? No doubt a scientist could answer it with some physiological or psychological explanation, but I must abide by my own storytelling mode. Again, as with Professor Fry's aged black informants, I believe that Henry Reed could play the fiddle despite his infirmities because that art, ingrained into him since early childhood, occupied some deeper stratum of his psyche where palsy held no sway. The art was of a characteristic regional style, built of an elaborate musical grammar of finger patterns and bowing patterns. These patterns, and the creative use of them, were not simply a matter of conscious effort, but had been fully assimilated into his being since childhood. He no more reflected consciously about how to move his bow arm in the classic patterns of his region than he thought about where to put his tongue to make the letter *t*. Hence his art was largely exempted from the deterioration that arises from the failure of the physical body to carry out the dictates of the conscious will.

The moral of this story, too, is that folk arts comprise a deep and potent strain in the human psyche: *deep,* because folk arts express fully assimilated cultural patterns and social values for people, going beyond the level of conscious, personal cultural acquisition to a level of shared expressive identity; *potent,* because though the expressive strain in all of us may lie fallow in alien or nonnurturing surroundings, it does not die but can be tapped again a half-century later to give vent to creative and expressive potentials we might never have imagined we had.

Folklife, then, if one is to believe the moral of these stories, offers us a special channel by which a wellspring of creativity may be tapped in old people. But we must be cautious here. Not just any folk art will do. The old woman in a Norwegian community in Kansas may have a tradition of fashioning exquisitely crafted woven hotpads or potholders, but it does not follow that we should set about mobilizing every rest home in the country toward the production of potholders. Nor do all old people need a little fiddle music on Saturday night to uplift their spirits and fire their imaginations.

Rather, experience with folklife teaches us to look for these creative wellsprings between the category of individual needs and personalities, on the one hand, and the category of national or universal patterns and habits, on the other. Tapping the creative potential of folk arts means developing a sensitivity to the variety of regional, ethnic, occupational, or religious traditions which have a special evocative potential for special groups of people. No formula will serve us well, for tapping folk arts means fundamentally drawing out special forms of expression people already possess, not laying on arts, forms, or programs they lack. Certain cultural professionals, like folklorists, specialize in studying these various artistic traditions in the United States, and many thoughtful and sensitive citizens sense the importance of folk cultural traditions in nurturing the creativity of the elderly. Turning that broad insight into useful programs and policies is no easy task, but it would be a welcome first step if specialists in aging and specialists in folk arts and folklife began trading thoughts and experiences, or even working together.

CREATIVITY AND THE RHYTHMS OF THE LIFE CYCLE

Many of America's finest folk artists are old people. In fact, many of the world's folk artists are old people. That statement might sound odd, or self-evident, or even silly, but it deserves a little reflection. I have often heard people express surprise that so many old folks do so many things so well. "Isn't it great that he can still play music!" "As old as she is, she still makes things for her grandchildren." "When he got going, he proved that he still was unsurpassed as a yarn spinner!" There seems to be an underlying presumption in all such remarks that one's peak in life and art of course comes earlier in life. Thereafter, whether the slope is gentle or precipitous, skill and creativity must gradually drain away. Hence the mild wonderment that "they can still do it."

It did not take me long working with folklife to realize what a seriously wrongheaded view of the world this was. Let me return to my experiences in the 1960s while visiting and recording traditional fiddlers in the upper South. My object was to document their art and to try to understand how that art related to their whole way of life. I was also learning to play the fiddle myself, and I must confess I was deeply moved by the beauty and thrilled by the excitement of learning the art from them. Thus I was a little surprised to hear from the old fiddlers I first encountered that several of them had stopped playing for twenty or thirty years, then begun again recently. Each had his reasons, of course. One quit because his wife could not stand the music. For another, the combined burdens of long work hours and raising a big family simply crowded the fiddle out. Yet another stopped playing for religious reasons. When three old men had told me such stories, the stories seemed to me to be simply personal accounts of particular lives. But by the time I had heard thirty versions of the story from fiddlers scattered across the Upper South, I began to realize that something bigger and more fundamental was going on. There was a larger rhythm to their life, and to their art, which was wholly at variance with my notions. If my mission had been to hunt out older fiddlers, I was not simply finding a few who still played. Rather, I was learning that old age was precisely when one played the fiddle.

The larger rhythm of fiddling in life, for these artists, was more or less as follows:

1. Age 7–15, learning to play
2. Age 15–30, learning the art

3. Age 30–55, the middle period
4. Age 55–90, the flowering of old age

These age brackets, to be sure, are loose and are provided only
to give a sense of a typical. But there is no question that the
pattern exists. Most traditional fiddlers in the upper South begin to play between the ages of seven and fifteen. A few musicians begin later, but it is a general rule in learning to play
the violin that the earlier one starts, the more likely it is that
one will become proficient. The first stage, then, is the stage
when the magic of music is first instilled and the fundamentals of the instrument are absorbed.

The second stage occurs during youth and early adulthood.
(In most cases it is early manhood, since traditional fiddling in
the United States has historically been the province of males.)
During this period the youth moves from learning the fundamentals to a vigorous and energetic assimilation of the art in
its finer points, using older players as models and tapping the
energies of fellow musicians in his peer group for reinforcement. The third stage, which I refer to above as the "middle
period," is a stage during which many fiddlers allow their ar-
tistry to go fallow. Some players continue through the middle
years of life without their musical participation abating, but
they are often those whose musicianship has earned them a
special designation within the community—in the old days,
say, the fiddler whom everybody calls for at community
dances, or in contemporary times the fiddler who plays in a
semiprofessional band. The middle period is characteristically
a stage of life where music is appreciated but pursued with
less energy than one's job, home, family, and other concerns.
The fiddle, one might say, plays second fiddle.

Finally, the fourth stage is the flowering of old age, often
fostered by semiretirement, the disburdening of the fiddler
from some of his responsibilities of the middle period, and the
arrival of grandchildren. During this stage many fiddlers
again take up the fiddle actively and regularly, get back into
practice, and take pleasure in sharing and imparting their art
to children and young people. They may in some instances acquire new styles, items of repertory, and techniques which are
in current favor. But the core of their artistic attention is ad-

dressed to the fundamental styles and repertories acquired during the second stage, a generation or two before. Thus the young fiddler of stage two becomes the "old-time fiddler" of stage four simply by returning energetically to what he once did.

Of all arts, folk arts are most intimately bound up with a way of life, and it is thus no surprise that the cycle of artistic expression melds with the larger rhythm of the life cycle. Of course, other arts may reveal a different life cycle from fiddling. One which is quite different, yet which clearly flowers in old age, is American folk painting. All of us recall Grandma Moses, and I well recall what a fuss was made of the fact that she started painting late in life. How extraordinary and unusual it seemed that, after living a full normal life, she should begin painting and prove to be so good and so productive in her old age! But in the last couple of decades specialists in folk art have uncovered many older women and men whose folk artistic development followed a similar pattern. Here again, then, we are not witnessing an unusual or quirky personal history, but a deeper cycle of art and life where old age is the *proper* time for creativity.

CREATIVE SYMBIOSIS BETWEEN OLD AND YOUNG

My final subject is the powerful *symbiotic* relationship between old people and young people. Some contemporary program planners working with the aged have, by luck or design, tapped the potential of this symbiosis. But I am not at all certain that they are aware how strong the special relationship is which binds together the elderly and the young in human society. One important form of this symbiotic principle is *grandparent education,* an ancient technique of cultural transmission in many cultures of the world that bestows on grandparents (or, by extension, the elderly in general) the special responsibility of educating children and imbuing them with the fundamental values of the culture. The principle has a certain timeless and universal efficacy, perhaps because it ensures that children can rebel against their parents without simultaneously rejecting the entirety of traditional knowledge and values. Grandparent education could be considered a fundamental social mechanism providing for both preservation and adaptation, both continuity and change. The principle could be illustrated by any number of stories involving American folklife and folk art, but I shall once again turn to my personal experience from the period when I embarked on my program of visiting and recording oldtime fiddlers in the Upper South.

I had played the violin myself since childhood, so in addition to studying, recording, and documenting these fiddlers as a young scholar, I was also relearning the instrument in their style as a young enthusiast. Though as a scholar one might be interested in documenting a wide spectrum of this sort of artistic expression, as an enthusiast I was inevitably drawn to certain fiddlers more than others. They all could teach me something, but the style and repertory of a few proved compelling enough to induce me to make many return visits. Henry Reed of Glen Lyn, Virginia, was one such artist. As I related earlier, he was in his eighties when we became acquainted, and he had plenty of leisure time to entertain me when I came calling. During my first visit with him, I recorded about forty tunes of his playing. Many of them were tunes I had never heard before, and it was clear from both his repertory and his intricate and complex style that he was an artist of the first order.

As soon as I could arrange it, I was back at his doorstep, tape recorder and fiddle in hand. Once again he welcomed me warmly and cordially. Once again I recorded a large batch of tunes, many of which I had never encountered, and once again I hesitatingly brought out my own fiddle to try and play along with him as occasion presented itself.

The third visit and the fourth visit followed the same pattern. Several weeks separated my visits, and during the interim I would often listen to the tapes at home and try to learn to play the pieces he played. By the fourth visit I suddenly became aware of a pattern. The first eight or ten tunes he played for me were tunes he had never played before. In the normal course of home fiddle playing, particularly when the occasions are separated by several weeks or months, one is likely to repeat a number of tunes one played the last time. Furthermore, it is very common for fiddlers to start out a session with a tune that is a perennial favorite of theirs, or a well-known favorite of the community's. Thus it began to dawn on me that there could be only one explanation of the fact that the first ten pieces he played were pieces he had never played for me before. The explanation was that he was actively conscious of his role as a teacher.

While I was away he must have been making mental notes of tunes as they occurred to him, reminding himself to be sure to play them for that young fellow when he came again. Not a word was spoken about this, but when I realized what was happening, I was deeply touched. First, it was a palpable reminder that in his eyes I was not simply documenting the music; rather, he saw me as a student or apprentice learning the music. So far as my personal yearnings were concerned, needless to say, he was right on the mark. Second, I came to see that those visits with Henry Reed, which had become so important to me as an aspiring young fiddler, were in their way just as important to him as an aging master. His sons and daughters were all quite musical, but none had taken up the fiddle— perhaps, as is often the case, because as their father he was a bit too close for direct emulation. I thus became a sort of foster-grandson, artistically speaking. Instead of documenting the process of folk culture, I found myself ineluctably drawn into participating in the process. It takes nothing away from his gift to me to say that it was as important for him to be able to give as for me to be able to receive.

My visits with Henry Reed, then, are a perfect example of the symbiosis between old people and young people for which a folk art can serve as the catalyst. More specifically, the relationship illustrates the principle of "grandparent education" through which cultural values can be passed along through time, even with the skipping of generations. Henry Reed himself as a youth learned from old men, and I often think as I play certain tunes he taught me that they are from, say, Quincy Dillion, a fiddler who was born in the early years of the nineteenth century. Though, in the usual manner of speaking, many generations and a sea of social change separate me from the early nineteenth century, in another sense I am only once removed through Henry Reed.

CONCLUSION

Let me try to summarize my conclusions, if "conclusions" is the appropriate term for a storytelling session. First, folklife is an expressive touchstone that can tap the deepest wellspring of human creativity. For the elderly it thus offers an important channel for spiritual nourishment at the deepest level. Second, folk artistic expression not only survives into old age, but often flowers in old age in obedience to profound cultural rhythms in the cycle of human life. Third, folklife builds ties between the old and the young, wherein the creativity in both is encouraged and enhanced by symbiotic cultural exchange. This exchange, which I have referred to as "grandparent education," is education in the most serious sense, in that it ensures both continuity and creativity in the transmission of culture through time.

Pondering these three conclusions emboldens me to offer a fourth. If folk arts and folklife offer us special insights into creativity and aging, they also caution us against treating creativity and aging in too compartmentalized a fashion. My relationship with Henry Reed was good for him, and good for me as well. I thus cannot help thinking that, though it can be helpful to ponder policies or programs for the elderly, or for the young, ultimately both the elderly and the young will profit most from a broad and informed approach to culture designed for the cultural nourishment of us all.

REFERENCE

Fry, Gladys-Marie. 1975. *Nightriders in Black Folk History*. Knoxville, Tennessee: University of Tennessee Press.

8 A PERFORMER'S PERSPECTIVE

James A. Standifer

During an interview in his home in 1974, Eubie Blake, a well-known and respected musician now in his ninety-eighth year, made an eloquent charge to me that resulted in my research on creativity among elderly black musicians. He said: "Too few writers and so-called researchers on black music are taking the trouble to consult with the very individuals who lived and made black music history." Those who have interviewed them, he continued, have frequently exploited them financially, causing distrust and suspicion. But, he said, "The researcher truly dedicated to black music experience should take hold of this work and get on with it, because with each passing day, we lose irreplaceable resources for this valuable information." Almost as an afterthought, Eubie shouted: "And this work should be done by black boys like you! What's the matter with y'all?"

I could not answer Eubie at that time, but I can say that he is responsible for much of the research I do these days. Supported by a grant from the National Endowment for the Humanities, I spent the last year researching the creative musical output of more than thirty elderly black musicians, ranging in age from sixty-three to ninety-eight. I visited the homes and workplaces of these artists, interviewed them, and

151

videotaped or audiotaped them talking and performing. I also talked with many individuals close to each of the artists.

In addition to interviewing artists such as Eubie, Alberta Hunter, Sippie Wallace, Andy Kirk, and others, I did some research on creativity, aging, and musical performance. Eubie was right: there has been an appalling lack of scholarly, sensitive research on elderly black musicians in particular, and on creative musical performance and longevity in general. With a view to redressing some of this neglect, this chapter will touch on both subjects.

Among the studies of creativity and aging, the most often cited include studies by Harvey C. Lehman (1953), Wayne Dennis (1966), R.N. Butler (1967), John A.B. McLeish (1976), and E.P. Torrance (1977). Most of these focus on quantitative measures of creative output versus age. Only "classical" artists are included in the musician list; moreover, with the notable exception of discussions by John McLeish, none of these studies include artists of black music. While some much-needed insight has been gained from these authors, the relevance of most proved problematic. For example, as far as I can determine, most of the research was conducted on white populations, and for the most part on persons who have long since died. Few glimpses of the viewpoints of the creators themselves are provided. In fact, the most cited studies (Dennis 1966; Lehman 1953) show the authors going to great lengths to have others act as resource banks and contribute to decisionmaking regarding major performances of persons who are dead. Lehman, for example, uses historians, panels of judges, an encyclopedia, dictionaries of biography, histories of art, lists of best-known works, and the like to assemble age data for creative contributions of highest merit in the lives of selected individuals.

Another contributor and keynote speaker for this series, John McLeish, has given an interesting assessment of Lehman's study, *Age and Achievement,* providing strong reinforcement for the basic direction of my research. He writes:

> The very people who should perhaps know more than anyone else about the peaks and valleys, the ebbs and flows of their own creative life—the creators themselves—never get a chance to speak at

all. Our judgments of when the writers, scientists, inventors, painters, athletes, musicians, and statesmen achieved the "peak" of creative action are left to armies of ghostly commentators and critics or to paragraph writers in encyclopedias. Their verdicts are marshalled and counted by anonymous scrutineers in a healthy democratic exercise culminating in the placing of the masterwork in its appropriate half-decade for charting (1976, p. 151).

Lehman demonstrated, as others in the field have done, that levels of achievement across fields are apt to vary widely. He left little question that there is a definite relationship between age and total productivity that, on the whole, tends to fall off with increasing years (Roe 1972). However, this is a purely quantitative approach to creativity, though Lehman would deny this, maintaining that he has selected the "best" works of artists for inclusion in his studies.

Lehman's lists of peak ages of artists (nearly all in their twenties and thirties) contribute to, rather than diminish, the negative vision our society has about the value and potential of adults in their later years. As if to soften the impact of his data, the author gives the following comment regarding total absolute output beyond the thirties, in a reply to one of the many critiques of his study: "The median chronologic ages in (the) tables reveal that (roughly) about half of the total of the 'most significant' creative contributions appear beyond age forty" (Lehman 1956).

For my purposes, the approach of Lehman and others has another important weakness: the most significant contributions studied were fixed objects—even icons. Insofar as black music and the elderly black musician are concerned (with perhaps the notable exception of black artists of "classical" or Western art music), such a conceptualization seems inappropriate, even antiaesthetic. The creative object studied has been removed from the basic realities of life and from the process that reflects those realities, namely the process of creating.

This leads us to two opposing conceptions of art: that art results from the operation of creating and that art is the operation of creating. I have placed black music in the latter category. In this study of creativity and the black elderly musician, black music is defined as music composed, arranged, or performed by blacks—musical behavior manifestly cultural in terms of experiences shared as a result of being black in America. It is music that includes many styles variously classified as blues, spirituals, gospels, ragtime, jazz, and more recently, rhythm and blues.

The forms of music associated with the musicians interviewed in my study are generally spontaneous and improvisatory. They are not fixed products in the same sense as the masterworks or peak achievements of classical musicians (e.g., symphonies, operas, chamber works). The great classics are honed and refined until a finished product results. In contrast, a fine jazz piece, blues, or gospel song grows and evolves before the audience, seeming to take on increasing spontaneous vitality (especially if the audience and performer are "in sync") as the music progresses. One performer offered this idea:

> There seems to be a mutual stroking process going on between me and what I'm creating. I'm often just as surprised and just as pleased as my listeners when I've had a particularly hot set. Sometimes I whisper to myself, "Man! that was a gas!" But there's a problem, and it's kinda like sex (yes, Jim, we old folks still do it), I try again and again to reach that peak and, like sex, more often than not, I don't quite get there! Also, as I've grown older, those levels are fewer and fewer; I find it more and more difficult to do what my mind tells me to do. . . .

"I guess that too," he said smiling, "is like sex."

In my study, these forms of music are examined as dynamic behavior inextricably tied to the performance technique and skill of black musicians performing black music. The manifestations of these behaviors—these musics—are viewed as the constantly changing and refreshed recreated work of the Louis Armstrongs, the Ella Fitzgeralds, the Sallie Martins, the Mahalia Jacksons, the Alberta Hunters, the Sippie Wallaces, the Edith Wilsons. The highly creative process and spontaneous behavior add up to a great deal more than any finished product; many of those interviewed felt that anything short of an examination of and active involvement—through clapping, moving, singing, and the like—in the experience of black music are apt to produce an erroneous view of the music.

Jimmy Stewart, a controversial writer on the black aesthetic, underlines this idea that the dynamic process in black music is immensely more important than the result. He writes:

What results therefrom is merely the momentary residue of that operation—a perishable object and nothing more, and anything else you might imbue it with (which the white aesthetic purports to do) is nothing else but mummification. The point is—and this is the crux of our two opposing conceptions of being—that the imperishability of creation is not in what is created, is not in the art product, is not in the thing as it exists as an object, but in the procedure of its becoming what it is (Stewart 1971, p. 84).

This concept of musical behavior bespeaks action, freedom, confidence, risk taking, and life—how life actually feels and moves. If we accept this proposition, then our task is clear: we must study the performance of these musical forms (preferably by the musicians themselves) and the life histories of the individual performers or musicians in question. We must also develop a profile of the various phases of the musicians' performance styles and practices, gleaned from personal observations and from views of the artists' most discerning biographers.

The individuals interviewed in my study differ widely in their degree of eminence and in the degree to which they are currently involved in their art. Some, like Eubie Blake or Alberta Hunter, are involved in almost a full rebirth of their commercially successful years; others perform only occasionally. In addition to videotaping interviews, I read biographies, talked with road managers, accompanists, or others, and examined as many recorded samples of the artists' work as possible. As might be expected, few of the artists are served well by the somewhat primitive recording techniques of the early days.

Much consideration was given to some of the dangers and limitations of this type of research. I was forewarned by many critics of oral histories, and my views about the worth of material gleaned from the interviews are probably kept in perspective by such criticisms. One scholar using this approach with bluesmen points out:

Materials gained in interviews have been severely criticized by some scholars. The musician is seen as an inarticulate man who knows too little or jives too much. . . .
The co-cultural participant, with his special insight and appropriate responses is too burdened with emotional and psychological dependencies. Laboring under his experiences, he is unable to formulate any cut-and-dried, simple statements about the rules

governing his groups' behavior. He is too close to be objective. And finally, because of his vested interest, he is liable to emphasize a positive and partial view of his group (Pearson 1968, pp. 221–222).

I disagree with such a statement and believe strongly in the artist's ability to interpret his own work. It is, of course, necessary to be aware of some of the pitfalls. Sharp awareness is perhaps the investigator's greatest protection here. I tried in a variety of ways to free informants from stock answers or from bringing to the interview situation a stage role or mask assumed to conform to their perceptions of my expectations. As Pearson has noted of bluesmen, "They have developed a predictive awareness of the questions that will be asked and how best to respond in keeping with their social identity as musicians. Repetition in questioning, involving topics which have come to define the blues artist's role, pressure the artist to organize his life according to these clichés" (pp. 214–215). To help avoid this limitation in oral testimonies, I informed the subjects (in different language, of course) that it is well documented that "a major source of error and falsification (in the interview process) is the influence exerted in the contents of a testimony by the function of the testimony and the purpose of the informant" (Vansina 1965, p. 95).

The musicians all readily agreed to cooperate and volunteered the fact that they and other musicians had victimized some interviewers by using their past experiences and understanding of these interviewers' beliefs about the informant and his art to their advantage. They emphasized that the artist knows that oral statements regarding his performance and life are apt to find their way into the media; almost inadvertently, he uses the opportunity to promote himself. An example of the kind of response I received to my preinterview plea for candor is this, provided by one eighty-two-year-old female blues singer:

> Honey, at my age, I figure I ain't got the *time* or the *need* to con anybody about anything. Even when I perform, I don't fear or expect anything. I just do what I do, and they love me. Now death is coming someday, and I can't get too excited about that. But I knows that it is one disease that there ain't no cure for. So I stays

ready. I think most old folks do. I live humble and try to be honest in all things.

In preparing to interview these musicians about creativity and aging, I felt that I needed a definition of creativity that would encompass a wide range of activities. Papers by Romaniuk (1979) and Parnes (1972) formed the basis for my own study's behavioral definition of creativity. Briefly, these authors define creativity as an openness to experience and change. They point out that creative behavior demonstrates both uniqueness and value to the community at large and to the individual. Specifically, Romaniuk suggests two basic components in creativity: first, one's past and current knowledge and experience as the raw material for creative activity; and second, one's ability to stimulate and recombine that knowledge and experience into some unique or exceptional form. Abraham Maslow's discussion of creativity (1954) also has relevance here. He says that while creativity is a

potentiality given to all human beings at birth, most people lose it as they become encultured. But, creativity may be renewed or recovered later in life. Additionally, it need not manifest itself in the usual artistic endeavors, it may be much more humble. It is as if this special type of creativeness being an expression of healthy personality, is projected out upon the world or touches whatever activity the person is engaged in (p. 223).

The musicians interviewed in my study are all enormously creative people who exemplify these definitions in their lives. They had many interesting ideas and feelings about how aging had affected their art. As I discuss their comments, it should be remembered that this is a very diverse group. I interviewed singers, dancers, songwriters, and instrumentalists, all of whom had their own unique perspectives on the subject at hand. The group included very old, relatively uneducated blues musicians, as well as younger, highly educated people such as Ann Brown. While Brown (the first Bess of *Porgy and Bess*) lives prosperously in Norway, earning her living as a teacher and writer, others live in very modest housing in Chicago, New York, Detroit, and Dallas and are still struggling to support themselves.

As a group, however, they felt that to grow with grace and fulfillment, especially as a performer, is to adjust one's performance and attitudes to the ostensibly inevitable physical and social changes that are concomitant with the normal period of adult life we refer to as aging. You will note that the word "adjust" rather than "accept" is used here in reference to these changes. None of the individuals indicated that they were willing, or even able, to simply accept what life "dished out" without putting up a fight. All agreed, however, that one must adjust daily if one is fortunate enough to live a longer-than-average life, and if one desires to hold on to that gift of longevity.

There was another theme that persisted throughout the conversations and interviews. They all felt that elderly black musicians share a common experience of hardship that has made them tough and taught them that in order to survive and be effective, not only did they have to be creative in dealing with the usual problems associated with their careers, they also had to use talent to cope with growing old, and being poor and black in America. This toughness, this strength, is probably typical of most performers who survive the ravages and discipline of their profession and who use their creative powers in their later years to preserve their image. No one should forget, they said, that elderly blacks have been "moulded" and "programmed" by a society that required them to be creative. They dealt with "a lot of stupidness" that was different from that normally experienced by other artists because of a fixed and conspicuous racial and musical identity. Indeed, there is no need to recount the problems suffered by blacks fifty or sixty years ago.

I asked Eubie Blake, Jester Hairston, and others why they and other blacks of the time allowed themselves and their talents to be used in so many demeaning and racist situations in the early days of black music and theater. Why did they permit their music to be published with terrible caricatures of blacks on the cover, write and perform countless Jim Crow sequences, and so on? Eubie's blunt answer: "First, probably to eat ... to be heard; mostly, so that you and others like you could be at the University of Michigan doing the wonderful things you're now doing!"

Jester Hairston, a composer, conductor, and actor, who played the very proper Henry Van Porter on the radio and TV versions of "Amos 'n Andy," and starred in the TV series "That's My Mamma," answered in a similar way. He added:

> There are lean times between paychecks as a musician. To take up the slack, I tried acting. I played in all of the old Tarzan (Johnny Weismuller) pictures. You can find me running around naked with rings in my nose and a spear in my hand. And, as you can see, I am already black as a biscuit. But would you believe I permitted them to paint me even darker so that I would have a "purplish glow" to my skin? Now ain't that a trip? But I ate, . . . raised a family, and all the while I was also doing what I *really* love: making music . . . especially black spirituals. By the way, I still get checks from residuals for those old Tarzan movies. I use them to help young blacks avoid the problems other blacks and I faced years ago.

One of those who endured her share of hardships but retained her charm and naturalness into her eighties is Edith Wilson, a blues singer who died in 1981. She had lived in what she called "a scuzzy part of South Chicago" for more than thirty years, and her home was completely decorated with vintage 1920s and 1930s furnishings. While she said that she wrote more songs in old age, she also returned to performing occasionally. Edith's most recent triumph took place during the summer of 1980 on Broadway. She starred in *Black Broadway*, along with several elderly blacks, including John Bubbles, Honi Coles, and Bobby Short. Her accompanist when she performed was usually Eureal "Lil" brother Montgomery, who lived only minutes from her and talked with her almost daily. I asked Miz Wilson, "Is your singing as good now as it was when you were in your prime?" Her quick reply: "Can you cut the mustard like you did when you were a teenager?" "Sometimes," I happily replied. "Then that's your answer," she said.

In the course of the interview Miz Wilson sang a song she wrote about old people, which she specifically tailored to her eighty-year-old voice. Called "Twiddling Your Thumbs," the lyrics are:

> There was a time so I've been told
> you was done when you grow old.

And that talk is now passé
'cause old folks have a ball today.

They have music, they have dancin',
winin', dinin', and romancin'.

They're always movin' to keep
from twiddling their thumbs.

They play golf and they fly planes
never have any aches or pains.

Just keep on movin' to keep
from twiddling their thumbs.

Now grandma and grandpa used to bunny
    hug,
now grandma holds a real cool cat and
grandpa sure can cut a rug.

Grandma goes to church on Sunday,
grandpa finds him a dice game on Monday.

Always movin' to keep from twiddling their
    thumbs.

Many of the performers I interviewed have, like Edith Wilson and Eubie Blake, returned to performing, as old musical styles came back into vogue. Alberta Hunter is perhaps a classic example. After walking away from her singing career in her fifties, she returned to school, received a practical nursing degree, and worked in a hospital until a couple of years ago, when Barney Josephson, owner of The Cookery in New York City, sought her out to perform in his club. Her first instinct, she says, was to refuse because she didn't want "to cut a hog" (to mess up) at age eighty. However, she accepted and has been performing around the country ever since.

Mary Lou Williams, a pianist, became frustrated by the greed in the music business and quit in 1954. For fifteen years she kept busy in church activities, until a Jesuit priest convinced her to return to performing. At age seventy, she was artist-in-residence at Duke University, and until her death in 1981 performed regularly throughout the world.

Sippie Wallace also quit performing in middle age, and spent nearly forty years as organist, singer, and choir director at the Leland Baptist Church in Detroit. In 1965 a local blues buff found Sippie and convinced her to return to the stage, and like the others, she has been singing ever since.

Obviously, none of these performers has lost creativity in old age. While all have had to adjust their performing styles to some extent, they are now much sought after and well respected. Other people whom I interviewed have found other outlets for their creative talents as they have aged. Anne Brown has lived in Norway for thirty years. Not only does she speak and write fluent Norwegian, but she teaches singing and drama at the National Theatre in Oslo. This is her comment about creativity and aging:

> When I was young, we used to hear the expression very often that enough is not sufficient. You must be very, very good—and then give more! As I've grown older, this statement rings truer and truer.
>
> The trend today is to do your thing as well as you can and don't bother about the rest. That's not my idea. I suppose I'm old-fashioned, but I think you should give everything you've got but hold tenaciously to your beliefs and integrity as a human being. I firmly believe that if you're going to be an artist and have real greatness as your goal, you *must* feed and nurture your gift of creativity in this way. Like a plant that's properly fed in its early period, your gift of creativity will strive and serve you for a very long while. It may wither a bit, but the right kind of environment will make it return as fresh as ever!

Andy Kirk, the famous band leader of the Twelve Clouds of Joy Band, dropped out of sight for years. Obviously wishing to stay in touch with the musical world, he now at age eighty-two works at a musicians' union, Local 802 in New York City.

Perhaps the most articulate statement about the creative process as it relates to aging emerged in my interview with Katherine Dunham. Now in her sixties, this internationally known dancer and choreographer is artist-in-residence at Southern Illinois University. Her statement sums up much of what the others indicated in various ways, and provides a fitting close to this discussion:

> Well, [as I age] I have certainly been able to recognize physical limitations, but I recognized them also while I was performing. I had certain limitations that made me change the choreography for myself or made me more interested in choreography only, rather than dancing. I have never been a person who wanted to just dance. I have always been interested in developing people and developing for other people, so I find age has nothing to do with this. I find also that I have more time to decide whether or not I am going to be a writer; I have done a great deal of writing. Maybe I'll do some more. I certainly hope so. . . . I would say that I find more possibility to express what I want to do, which is develop people and help humans to become secure in themselves and less alienated. I find that is a great challenge here, one that goes on endlessly.
>
> It is hard to convince an individual who is going to the top that they should be very careful about the possibilities of aging. Now I am thinking about physical aging. A violin player has to be careful of his hands. A dancer is in a total production; a dancer has to be careful of everything, a finger, a toe, or this or that or the other. So a dancer is constantly aware of his body, and I would say: continue this awareness. Do not think you are going to go on forever, because you are not. And begin to plan on this or that or the other; begin thinking of something else.
>
> And so, many dancers paint. I used to paint. I started again recently. Start something else that makes use of your creative ability, because if you do not you will die inside as a person. [Standifer: So you are saying to redirect your energies?] Yes. A creative person has to create. It does not really matter what you create, you know. If such a dancer wanted to go out and build catcus gardens where he could, in Mexico, let him do that, but something that is creative has to go on!

REFERENCES

Butler, R.N. 1967. "The Destiny of Creativity in Later Life: Studies of Creative People and the Creative Process." *Psychodynamic Studies on Aging: Creativity, Reminiscing, and Dying*, edited by S. Levin and R.J. Kahana. New York: International Universities Press.

Dennis, Wayne. 1966. "Creative Productivity between the Ages of 20 and 80 Years." *Journal of Gerontology* 21.

Lehman, Harvey C. 1953. *Age and Achievement*. Princeton, N.J.: Princeton University Press.

Lehman, Harvey C. 1956. "Reply to Dennis' Critique of *Age and Achievement*." *Jounal of Gerontology*, 2:333–337.

McLeish, John A.B. 1976. *The Ulyssean Adult: Creativity in the Middle and Later Years*. New York: McGraw-Hill Ryerson Ltd.

Maslow, Abraham. 1954. *Motivation and Personality*. New York: Harper and Row.

Parnes, Sidney J. 1972. "Programming Creative Behavior." *Climate for Creativity*, edited by Calvin W. Taylor, pp. 193–227. New York: Pergamon Press.

Pearson, Barry Lee. 1968. *"The Life Story of the Blues Musician: An Analysis of the Traditions of Oral Self-Portrayal."* Ph.D. dissertation, Indiana University.

Roe, Anne. 1972. "Maintenance of Creative Output through the Years." In *Climate for Creativity*, edited by Calvin W. Taylor, pp. 167–91. New York: Pergamon Press.

Romaniuk, Jean Gasen. 1979. "Designing Creative Thinking Workshops for Older Adults." Paper presented at the fifth Annual Meeting of the Association for Gerontology and Higher Education, Washington, D.C., March 8–9.

Stewart, Jimmy. 1971. "Introduction to Black Aesthetics in Music." In *The Black Aesthetic*, edited by Addison Gayle, Jr., pp. 81–96. Garden City, N.Y.: Doubleday & Co., Inc.

Torrance, E.P. 1977. "Creativity and the Older Adult." In *Environment, Creativity, and Aging: Proceedings of the Fourth Annual Georgia Conference on Aging*. Athens, Ga.: University of Georgia Center for Continuing Education.

Vansina, Jan. 1965. *Oral Tradition: A Study in Historical Methodology*, translated by H.M. Wright. Chicago: Aldine Publishing Company.

III

UNIVERSITY OF SOUTHERN CALIFORNIA A TRIBUTE TO LONGEVITY

INTRODUCTION

James E. Birren

Among the most significant human developments in this century is the dramatic lengthening of the average span of life; in fact, on average, more has been added to the length of life in this century than was added from prehistoric times up to the last century. In 1900, the average family disintegrated with the death of one of the parents before the last child left home. The existence of unwanted orphans in society was a grave social problem. Miraculously, as people are living longer there are now not enough children available for adoption. Society has correctly shifted its focus from the child and the young nuclear family to the mature family. In a broad sense we are now entering the phase of the "adult society." In response to this new social emphasis brought about by increased longevity, the chapters in this part look at various implications of aging for individuals and for society.

Since the hereditary aspects of aging are among the most fundamental of biological phenomena, it is entirely appropriate to have a paper by George M. Martin, "A Genetic and Evolutionary Perspective on Aging and Longevity." If we are to reduce some of the liabilities of old age in humans, he points out, we must understand what aspects of biological aging we share with other species of animals and thereby gain valuable insight into the evolution of aging. It would be a tremendous step forward if we could study the vital biological processes of aging in selected small organisms whose life spans are but a few days. What is it that changes in short-lived cells as they grow old that makes them more susceptible to disease and the inability to maintain vital processes?

There is most likely no single lethal gene whose action determines how long we will live. According to George Martin, perhaps hundreds or thousands of genes may be involved in the acceleration or deceleration of aging. Much of what we need to know about aging requires advances in basic genetic knowledge, but at the same time the study of age-related genetic diseases can offer "windows" through which to view the fundamentals of genetic action in aging. Unfortunately, for such aspects of human suffering as senile dementia, progress is too slow for our patience. But we must remember that aging has been long in evolution, and despite our impatience, the secrets of aging may not yield quickly to research.

E.J. Masoro further explores the topic of longevity in his chapter on nutrition and aging. He develops for us the important point that food restriction slows the rate of aging in animals, and presumably in human populations as well. One must make the distinction here between a nutritionally adequate or balanced diet and one which is qualitatively deficient. The major point is that if animals are allowed to eat as much as they like of a balanced diet, they do not live as long as animals whose food intake is restricted. Of great importance is the finding that food restriction delays the onset of a wide range of age-related diseases in mice and rats. To this extent it is a general factor, not specific to a particular disease.

As yet, science has not pointed out the mechanisms by which dietary restriction brings about its influence on length of life. However, thoughtful people may well find it wise to voluntarily restrict their appetite and their food intake—to consider not only what they eat but also how much they eat—as knowledge advances about precisely how the beneficial effect is brought about.

Given the fact that in this century the average life expectancy of humankind has so dramatically increased, it is not surprising that we have become involved in moral and ethical issues about the right to life. In his chapter, John B. Orr considers the moral issues underlying the topics of aging, death, and the search by contemporary science for the secrets of longevity. He asserts that "people have the right to seek the longest life possible for themselves and their loved ones within a social system where reasonable opportunities to enhance the possibility for a long life have been fairly allocated within the population." However, he points out that the benefits of research and technology are not always equally distributed in the population. At the present time, mortality rates over most of the life span are significantly higher for the lower socioeconomic groups than for the economically favored. In a variety of ways, the better educated appear to be favored in the race through life.

Toward the end of a life, the question often arises as to how long existence should reasonably be prolonged if there is no consciousness or awareness and no prospect for the recovery of function. As more of us live to the later years, the issue of the right to die, in contrast with the right to live, will assume increasing importance. John Orr appropriately points out that a long life is not the same thing as a full life. In fact, current research tends to bear out the idea that long lives and full ones are more common today than in the past. In earlier generations, when we had frequent residual consequences of infectious diseases, paradoxically the burden of disability could last much longer than it does now in a population that is living significantly longer. Nevertheless at some point the question comes up about "the need for a good death." It is here where the humanities and those scholars who have thoughtfully considered issues of human life can contribute to our well-being. There is nothing in the fact of increasing longevity that justifies a preoccupation with death—rather, a good death at the end of a "well-crafted life" can be a celebration of life itself.

9 A GENETIC AND EVOLUTIONARY PERSPECTIVE ON AGING AND LONGEVITY

George M. Martin

Recently I had the great privilege of spending a sabbatical period of research at the Sir William Dunn School of Pathology at Oxford University, where penicillin was first isolated, characterized, and proved to be highly efficacious for treating a variety of bacterial infections. That accomplishment, like so many triumphs of modern medicine, has led to substantial increases in the average life span in human populations throughout the world. There is absolutely no evidence, however, that these scientific developments have altered in the slightest way the maximum life span of any population. According to Dr. Alex Comfort's careful review of the literature (1979), the maximum *fully authenticated* longevity for man is 113 years and 100 days, a record achieved by Pierre Joubert, a French Canadian who was born in 1701 and who died in 1814. So far as is known, he did this without the benefit of supplementary vitamin E, and quite possibly, despite the ingestion of generous quantities of wine, which I imagine was routinely prescribed for those harsh Quebec winters.

Maximum potential longevity is quite clearly a constitutional feature of the organism, written in the message of the genes. Like alterations in morphology, number and types of chromosomes, rates of development, and age of onset of puber-

171

ty, longevity is a manifestation of speciation—that genetically mediated process by which a new and distinctive group of organisms appears, whose members generally reproduce exclusively among themselves. Within mammalian species, there is a fortyfold to fiftyfold range in maximum life span. Reproducible differences in life tables can be demonstrated among laboratory animals that are somewhat related taxonomically and that are about the same size and general appearance. For example, under virtually identical laboratory conditions, the ordinary house mouse, *Mus musculus,* has a maximum life span of about three to four years, whereas the white-footed deer mouse, *Peromyscus leucopus,* has a maximum life span of about eight years (Sacher and Hart 1978).

Such comparative gerontology is a potentially powerful tool with which to search for fundamental biochemical genetic mechanisms of aging. The major focus of this chapter, however, will be on our own species, *Homo sapiens.* We are characterized by an extraordinary degree of genetic heterogeneity. Except for identical twins, no two individuals on the face of the earth are genetically identical.

Genes are segments of the viscous polymer DNA (deoxyribonucleic acid), which is located in the nuclei of our cells in the form of twenty-three pairs of chromosomes, one set having been inherited from each of our parents. Chromosomes, unlike genes, can be seen with the ordinary light microscope, and so it is comparatively easy to examine suitably prepared cells (such as those from the blood) of large numbers of individuals. Such surveys of living newborn infants have revealed frequencies of grossly abnormal chromosome sets ranging from 0.60 to 0.73 percent (Buckton et al. 1980). It is likely that more sensitive methods of examination will reveal even higher frequencies of abnormalities, so that one can conservatively estimate that one in a hundred live newborn infants bear such grossly abnormal karyotypes. This figure excludes more subtle alterations, which occur with considerably higher frequencies and which are called structural heteromorphisms.

An example of a structural heteromorphism is the considerable variation that exists in special regions associated with five pairs of human chromosomes, numbers 13, 14, 15, 21, and 22 (Evans, Buckland, and Pardue 1974; Jacobs 1977). These regions are called nucleolar organizers, and they carry copies for the genes that code for two special classes of RNA (ribonucleic acid) molecules. In turn, these RNA molecules are essential for the cell to construct numerous submicroscopic bodies called ribosomes, little factories that manufacture all of the cell's proteins. Strehler (1980) has done some very interesting experiments which indicate that there may be loss or masking of these genes in several tissues of humans and dogs as they age. If the extent of such loss can significantly diminish the cells' ability to produce proteins in the face of various injuries—for example, those resulting from coronary artery disease and poor blood flow to the heart muscle cells—then it would certainly be advantageous to start out life with some extra copies!

Most genes code for molecules of protein. We attribute our biochemical individuality mainly to slight variations in the structure and function of numerous proteins, including thousands of enzymes whose job it is to greatly speed up specific chemical reactions throughout the body. By subjecting such enzymes to an electrical field, one can detect single-charge differences in the molecule, alterations that result from certain variations in the genetic code within the DNA molecule. After such electrophoretic separations, one can specifically identify many types of enzymes by using special stains. When such studies are carried out on large populations of normal subjects, it is found that some 28 percent of the genes controlling the structure of such enzymes are polymorphic in that they code for variants of comparatively high frequency—arbitrarily defined by human geneticists as frequencies of the genes equal to or greater than 1 percent (Harris and Hopkinson 1972). This is clearly a minimum estimate of the extent of genetically controlled enzymatic variation, since the study excluded certain variants that did not display an electrical charge difference.

Immunological methods have also been used to define genetic polymorphisms in humans, since antibodies can detect very subtle alterations in the structure of proteins. Scientists throughout the world have used such immunological probes to determine the number of variant genes, or alleles, at each of four subloci within a rather large gene cluster in humans called HL-A, because they are antigens (A) mainly studied in human leukocytes (HL), or white blood cells. These antigenic proteins sit on the surfaces of virtually all cell types and are thought to play crucial roles in the regulation of various cell-to-cell interactions. They play an important role in the rejection of foreign tissues transplanted between genetically unrelated individuals, and in ways that are not yet understood, they serve as markers that predict which individuals are likely to develop such diseases as juvenile diabetes or certain forms of arthritis and hepatitis. From the number of gene variations at these four subloci so far discovered, it can be calculated that there are about a billion unique potential combinations of such genes (Bodmer et al. 1978; Bodmer 1980). If we consider that this is only one of the many thousands of such gene complexes and individual genes, the potential for genetic variation is truly remarkable.

Is it possible that, within this vast repertoire of genetic variation in humans, there are factors operating that might selectively modulate the rates of aging in various organs and tissues? In other words, are there varieties of genes that set the stage for more rapid decline in the structure and function of one individual's blood vessels, despite inheritance of other genes that encourage preservation of central nervous system functions? In another individual, might inheritance have set the stage for quite the reverse situation? To answer these questions, one would ideally like to carry out repeated quantitative physiological studies, starting from young adulthood and extending into old age, not only in selected individuals, but also in their entire pedigrees of blood relatives and in many other families as well. Such studies, of course, would be very expensive and time-consuming, and have in fact never been carried out. To do so we would have to have the sort of long-term support for scientific projects that rarely occurs in our society.

I have, however, approached the problem in a different way. Many genetic defects are not detectable at birth; in fact, some may not be manifested until well beyond sexual maturity. With this in mind, I systematically searched McKusick's comprehensive catalog of Mendelian inheritance in humans (1975) for genetic disorders characterized by an unusual susceptibility (either in terms of early onset, severity, or both) to a "senescent phenotype"—that is, conditions that the physician or pathologist would associate with aged people either in the clinics or on the autopsy table (Martin 1978).

Some of these features—graying of the hair, for example— are quite obvious to the layperson. Others of my selected markers of aging are well known only to the practicing pathologist and to biogerontologists, such as the accumulations within cells of yellow brown pigments called lipofuscins—oxidized, highly insoluble substances that gradually accumulate in special cell organelles as byproducts of metabolism. Still others of my markers of aging are more speculative in nature and were included because of certain experimental and theoretical lines of evidence—for example, possible defects in stem-cell proliferation.

Out of the total of 2,336 genetic loci, 162, or 6.9 percent, were judged to have potential relevance to the pathobiology of aging in that they revealed one or more aspects of the senescent phenotype. If we assume an upper limit for the number of genes in humans of 100,000, this would mean that almost 7,000 different genes might be playing a role in human aging. It is clear that there are complex polygenic controls of aging. Although no single gene can accelerate or retard all of the various features of aging, however, some abnormal genes do a pretty good job. I have referred to the genetic disorders that they produce as "segmental progeroid syndromes" (Martin 1978).

Werner's syndrome is one such disorder. Like most progeroid syndromes, it is fortunately quite rare, affecting about one out of a million people. The condition can be attributed to the affected individual's inheriting two copies of a single abnormal gene—one from the father and one from the mother. With the possible exception of premature graying of hair, the parents appear to live perfectly normal lives despite the fact that they each carry single copies of the abnormal gene. However, when two such carriers mate, as in some consanguineous marriages (first cousins, for example), with each pregnancy there is a one-in-four chance of producing a homozygotic offspring—that is, one carrying two copies of the abnormal gene.

Such affected individuals seem perfectly normal until adolescence, at which time they fail to undergo the spurt of growth normal during puberty. There then follows premature graying of the hair, loss of hair, thinning of the skin, the development of cataracts, diabetes, osteoporosis (softening of the bone), aging changes within the testes and ovary with loss of fertility, and several types of severe and premature arteriosclerosis or hardening of the arteries. More significantly, the patients suffer from severe and premature atherosclerosis, a disease that produces heart attacks with increasing frequency as humans age. Heart attacks, or myocardial infarctions, are a common cause of death in patients with Werner's syndrome, who die at an average age of forty-seven. Cancer is another common cause of death, particularly tumors derived from connective tissues, bone, fat, nerve sheaths, and smooth muscle, rather than tumors that derive from epithelial tissues.

Cultures of cells taken from the dermal layer of the skin of patients with Werner's syndrome have a markedly reduced life span as compared to age-matched controls. On a statistical basis they live some two to three standard deviations below the means of the control groups. Some years ago, Dr. Leonard Hayflick, working with Dr. Paul Moorhead at the Wistar Institute in Philadelphia, carefully measured the life span of normal cells taken from the lungs and skin of fetuses and adults and found that, in all cases, these cultures eventually stopped growing. In the best studied case, which involved cells grown from the lung of a fetus, the cultures doubled in population size from forty to sixty times before they became reproductively dead. Moreover, Hayflick demonstrated that cells from adults had considerably shorter life spans than cells from embryos. Our research and the research of Dr. Edward Schneider also confirmed this observation that the life span of such cultures is inversely related to the age of the donor. Many researchers around the world are therefore using such cultures as models of cellular aging, although it must be emphasized that such a model may only be relevant to one aspect of aging—namely, the limited replicative or reproductive life span of cells.

In Werner's syndrome, the cell culture observation has particular interest because it suggests that the fundamental biochemical genetic defect in this disorder is expressed in these cultured connective tissue cells. Such study thereby opens a door to the discovery of a specific enzyme defect governing a single chemical reaction that, when defective, results in such diverse and extremely important age-related pathologies as arteriosclerosis, cancer, diabetes, cataracts, osteoporosis, and skin atrophy.

In my systematic study of single-gene mutations that affect aging, I used as controls three relatively common human chromosomal abnormalities: (1) Klinefelter's syndrome, which occurs in men and results from one or more extra X chromosomes; (2) Turner's syndrome, which occurs in women and results from an absence of one of the two X chromosomes or from a deletion of part of one of the X chromosomes; and (3) Down's syndrome, which involves both men and women and results from an extra chromosome (a "trisomy") number 21, one of the five types of chromosomes that carry genes for the synthesis of ribosomal RNAs. As for the number of aging markers that these disorders display, each ranks within the top ten of 162 single-gene mutations of relevance to aging. In fact, the single genetic disorder with the greatest number of aging markers turned out to be one of the three chromosomal controls—Down's syndrome.

Most people are familiar with the characteristic facial appearance of young children with Down's syndrome, formerly called mongolism, but we are less familiar with older adult patients, in part because of their generally short life spans. Because of the profound mental deficiency of such patients, it took clinicians and pathologists a long time to realize that by the time such patients reach their thirties, they uniformly develop the classical features of senile dementia. These patients also show such features as accelerated autoimmunity (the presence in the serum of antibodies against one's own tissues), cataracts, premature graying or loss of hair, susceptibility to certain tumors (especially leukemias), and premature aging of the gonads. Moreover, while they suffer from certain degenerative diseases of small blood vessels (Reid and Maloney 1974), they may be comparatively resistant to the development of atherosclerosis (Murdoch et al. 1977).

To find accelerated aging in patients with these chromosomal imbalances has considerable theoretical interest. Unlike Werner's syndrome and the numerous other disorders that result from an abnormal gene, chromosomal syndromes such as Down's, Klinefelter's, and Turner's result from abnormal amounts of subsets of normal genes. Many geneticists believe that such gene imbalances result in great abnormalities in the regulation of gene expression. In other words, errors in the basic messages of the genes are not at fault; instead, there are probably abnormalities in such processes as the timing and coordination of gene action.

Are there other lines of evidence that might suggest the importance of gene regulation in determining life span and the onset of various signs and symptoms of aging? Some basic aspects of evolution in fact support this contention. In recent years, largely as a result of the research of Professor Alan Wilson and his colleagues (Wilson et al. 1977), it has become apparent that the rate at which new species are created has been much too rapid to be explained merely by the gradual accumulation of slight changes within individual genes. Since the great majority of genes control protein synthesis, a sample of such proteins from various species can determine how fast the genes have changed over the course of millions of years. The rates of change vary somewhat from protein to protein, but the changes are in general very slow and steady, serving as a sort of molecular clock. For example, the proteins of the chimpanzee are almost identical to those of a human, yet they are derived from species that diverted from one another some five million years ago. The differences between the anatomy and development of these two species is very considerable, however.

Studies of chromosomes, moreover, have suggested an alternative to this notion that evolution transpired through changes in the structure of proteins. When large groups of organisms were studied, it was discovered that there was an excellent correlation between the rates of chromosomal evolution within major groups of vertebrates and their rates of speciation (Bush et al. 1977). This is consistent with the notion that new species arise via rearrangements of already existing genes. Many biologists believe that such rearrangements may directly affect gene regulation, although certainly other interpretations are possible (Wilson et al. 1977).

Along with comparatively rapid rates of speciation among higher organisms, there developed comparatively rapid rates in the evolution of increased longevity. This phenomenon was documented by George Sacher (1970, 1975) and Richard Cutler (1975) in studies of the evolution of our hominid precursors. The cranial capacities and weights of these human precursors can be estimated from fossil remains. In turn, reasonable estimates of maximum longevity can be obtained by using formulas based on known correlations of longevity with brain size and body weight among living mammals. When one plots such data as the rate of change in maximum life span against time, a steady increase in maximum life span potential appears, reaching a maximum value of about 140 years per million years approximately 100,000 years ago (Cutler 1975).

If chromosomal rearrangements underlie such increases in longevity among higher primates, it is reasonable to ask which chromosomes were involved. The French cytogeneticist, Bernard Dutrillaux (1975) has created a flow diagram, based on the human chromosome numbering system, illustrating the sequence of chromosomal evolution from a common ancestor to the various branches leading to orangutans, gorillas, chimpanzees, and humans. The branch leading to humans evidently involved alterations in chromosome numbers 1, 2, 4, 9, and 18. It will, I think, be important for gerontologists to follow carefully the growing information on the human genetic map—that is, the localization of genes to specific sites on specific chromosomes—in order to determine which genes on these five chromosomes may be of special interest to their discipline. For example, there is already evidence that two genes occur in that set that have considerable relevance to a currently popular theory of aging: the intrinsic mutagenesis theory, most clearly enunciated by the distinguished Australian immunologist and Nobel laureate, Sir McFarlane Burnet (1974).

So far I have emphasized abnormal forms of genes, or mutations, that involve the germ line and are passed on from generation to generation. However, mutations can also directly affect the various types of cells in our body as we grow and age. Since these cells are part of the soma, that part of the body which is separate from the eggs and sperm and their precursor cells, the mutations are referred to as "somatic" cell mutations. The intrinsic mutagenesis hypothesis argues that the disabilities of old age result from accumulations of such somatic cell mutations. This immediately implicates several classes of genes as having exceptional significance for determining life span and modulating rates of aging.

One such set of genes are the enzymes called DNA polymerases. Their function is to replicate the genetic material—in other words, to make the required extra copies of genes when cells prepare for division. The actions of DNA polymerases are now being studied in the test tube in several laboratories. It turns out that, when copying DNA, these enzymes do in fact make occasional errors, so that the copies are not exact replicas of the original template strands of DNA. These methods therefore allow one to measure mutations in test tubes and to ask such basic questions as whether or not the enzymes from long-lived mice, such as the white-footed deer mouse, have higher fidelities of replication—make fewer mutations—than the enzymes from the short-lived house mouse. The intrinsic mutagenesis theory would predict that the polymerases for longer-lived species make fewer mistakes.

Another prediction of the intrinsic mutagenesis theory is that, given a comparable amount of damage to DNA, the somatic cells of long-lived animals can repair this damage more efficiently and completely than the cells of short-lived animals. There turn out to be a great number of enzymes, and therefore a great number of genes, that participate in the successful repair of various types of damage to DNA. One of these genes is probably located on chromosome 9. Could it be that, as a result of chromosomal evolution, this genetic locus became subject to more efficient regulation, leading to a more prompt and extensive repair of certain types of injuries to the genetic material in adult organisms?

There is no evidence on this point, but some interesting experiments by Hart and Setlow (1974) do suggest that longevity is related to a particular variety of DNA repair, called "UV-induced excision repair" (so called because the injurious agent is ultraviolet light and the repair involves a complicated cutting out and patching together of the damaged region). When cultured cells from mammalian species of contrasting longevities, ranging from the shrew to the elephant to humans, were damaged by irradiation with varying dosages of ultraviolet light, it was discovered that the rate and extent of repair directly correlated with the logarithms of the maximum life spans of the donor species. More recently, Drs. Ronald Hart and Katherine Hall set up cultures of cells from small biopsies of skin obtained from various species of monkeys and apes at the San Diego Zoo. Once again, they found that the longer the life span of the particular monkey, the more efficient was this particular type of DNA repair.

Similar types of positive correlative experimental results have been obtained by Dr. Arthur Schwartz of Temple University for the enzyme aryl hydrocarbon hydroxylase. Among the several functions of such enzymes is the ability to convert certain chemical compounds into highly reactive derivatives called epoxides, which can attack DNA and cause mutations. They can also cause cancer, presumably through their effects on DNA. In keeping with the intrinsic mutagenesis hypothesis, Schwartz found that cells from short-lived mammals were much more efficient in carrying out such chemical reactions than cells from long-lived mammals such as humans.

Can any of our human genetic diseases shed light on the intrinsic mutagenesis theory of aging? The type of DNA repair that Hart and Setlow measured in their studies with cells from many differentiated species of mammals is known to be defective in the great majority of patients with the clinical disorder xeroderma pigmentosum, a term of Greek origin referring to the dry and pigmented or freckled skin of such patients. Unfortunately, they suffer from much more dangerous lesions of the skin, including several types of cancers such as squamous cell carcinomas and basal cell carcinomas (two of the commonest types of cancer of the elderly), and malignant melanoma, a particularly virulent type that spreads widely throughout the body. All of the various skin pathologies seen in xeroderma pigmentosum appear on areas of the skin that are exposed to sunlight or other forms of ultraviolet light, including an abnormality called lentigo maligna, a precursor to one variety of malignant melanoma which is found almost entirely on the sun-exposed skins of the elderly population. We can conclude, therefore, that the genetically determined enzyme defect in these patients leads to premature aging of the skin.

But does it lead to premature aging of other organs? It turns out that there are at least six genetically distinctive subtypes of xeroderma pigmentosa, five of them with the classical UV-induced excision repair defect, and one with a poorly understood defect in what is called postreplication repair—that is, repair that may ensue after the DNA has completed its replication (Andrews, Barrett, and Robbins 1978). This can be demonstrated by a cell-genetic test called complementation analysis (Andrews et al. 1978). If cultured cells from a patient with the type A disease are fused to cells from patients with type B disease, or with any of the other types, the new hybrid cells now show a normal response to ultraviolet light. There is a mutual repair or complementation of their respective genetic defects, which can only come about if the respective gene products are nonidentical. When cells of type A are fused with cells from other patients with type A, there is no mutual correction; the hybrid cells behave just like the parent cells in that they remain very sensitive to the damaging effects of ultraviolet light.

Moreover, most patients from group A and all patients so far examined from group D have neurological abnormalities that some investigators believe to be due to the loss of cells in the brain—either central nervous system neurons or one or more of a variety of glial cells, so called because of the old belief that such cells constitute a sort of glue that gives the brain its structure. Although systematic, critical microscopic studies of the brains of these patients have yet to be carried out, I believe it is unlikely that the pathology will resemble what is found in aging brains. Certainly, the clinical picture is not what one would call dementia. Neurologically affected patients instead show retarded development with diminished intelligence, and they have defects in multiple portions of the nervous system (Robbins 1974). None of the other organ systems of the body, apart from the corneal and conjunctival portions of the eyes, show abnormalities. I would therefore conclude that the abnormal genes in xeroderma pigmentosum only mimic certain features of ordinary aging, mainly those related to the skin.

One other class of genetic loci is extremely important to those gerontologists who believe in the free radical theory of aging. Although the concept was first formalized by Dr. D. Harman in 1956, it was not until twelve years later, when two young biochemists at Duke University discovered a new class of enzymes called the superoxide dismutases (McCord and Fridovich 1968, 1969), that one could begin to consider seriously how specific genes might be important in the formulation of such a theory.

Free radicals are atoms or groups of atoms with one or more unshared electrons, and which are capable of forming chemical bonds with other atoms or molecules. They are highly reactive and usually very unstable. An example of free radical is the superoxide radical, O_2-, which results when ordinary molecular oxygen, O_2, is only partially reduced by causing it to lose only a single electron. Reduction by two electrons results in hydrogen peroxide, H_2O_2. Both products are highly reactive and potentially so toxic to living cells that nature has evolved, in all aerobic organisms—that is, all those that use oxygen for respiration—special enzymes that quickly neutralize or "scavenge" these dangerous byproducts of metabolism. The superoxide dismutases are clearly in the front line of such defense mechanisms: they speed up a chemical reaction forming hydrogen peroxide $(2O_2 + 2H^+ - H_2O_2 + O_2)$, which is then acted on by the enzyme catalase.

We can ask two questions about the significance of the superoxide dismutases to longevity. First, have the levels of activity risen in animal tissues along with the evolution of increasing maximum life spans among mammals and primates? Second, what can human genetic variants of the superoxide dismutases tell us about the biology of aging?

We have only very incomplete information relative to both questions. As regards the comparative gerontological approach, Dr. Richard Cutler and his colleagues (Tolmasoff, Ono, and Cutler 1980) do in fact have evidence that, in relation to animals' basic rate of metabolism of oxygen, the tissues of long-lived animals tend to have higher activities, presumably involving the major forms of this enzyme. As regards genetic variants, the population studies so far conducted suggest that the enzyme is so important for survival that few variations in its structure can be tolerated, at least those involving the active site, or critical portion of the molecule. A single variant has been found in northern Sweden (Beckman 1973; Beckman, Beckman, and Nilsson 1975), especially near the border with Finland, where it affects about 5 percent of the population (Beckman 1973). The affected people have Finnish surnames, so it is likely that the finding represents a contamination or an enrichment, depending on one's point of view, of Swedes by Finns. The enzyme activity of the purified enzyme was reduced only by about 15 percent in comparison with the usual enzyme (though there is always the worry that such artificial test tube assays do not accurately reflect what goes on in the cells of the body). Not much is known about how carriers of this presumably mildly defective enzyme fare into old age, since only a small number of people who have double doses of the abnormal gene have been studied to date. So far, they do not appear to be susceptible to any particular age-related disease—or to any other disease, for that matter.

In addition to asking about abnormal forms of the enzyme, we can ask about what happens to individuals with unusual amounts of the enzyme. Once again, we can learn something of importance from our patients with trisomy 21, or Down's syndrome. Since the gene for the major form of superoxide dismutase is located on chromosome 21, the cells from these patients, having three copies instead of the usual two copies of the gene, might be expected to have a 50 percent higher enzyme activity. This expectation has been verified by Dr. Charles Epstein and his colleagues at the University of California Medical Center at San Francisco (Feaster, Kwok, and Epstein 1977). Obviously, the extra dose of this valuable defense against the ravages of the superoxide free radical has not increased the life span of such patients, very few of whom survive into their sixties (Smith and Berg 1976), and all of whom develop senile dementia if they live much past age thirty. On the other hand, Down's syndrome patients may well be unusually resistant to atherosclerosis, the most important variety of hardening of the arteries (Murdoch et al. 1977). Could superoxide dismutases be especially important in protecting you and me from *that* particular age-related disorder? This is not a trivial question, as atherosclerosis is the most likely cause of disability and death for most of us.

As all these examples suggest, in order to understand how life span is determined, we must learn a great deal more about genetics. Evolutionary studies suggest that rearrangement of chromosomes was probably of crucial significance in the development of new species, including species with increasingly longer life spans. We suspect that these rearrangements affected the regulation or timing of gene action, but we know very little of the details of how this might be brought about.

In addition, by using our knowledge of the various human genetic disorders that can serve as probes for aspects of the aging process, we can make crude estimates of the number of genes involved in modulating aging rates, with the conclusion that no single gene can accelerate or decelerate all of the various aspects of aging, and that perhaps hundreds or thousands of genes are involved. It seems likely that, just as we are born as genetically unique individuals, we age in uniquely individual ways. While there are undoubtedly common denominators, the real challenge of gerontological science, in my view, is to discover exactly what mechanisms control those sometimes striking differences in susceptibility that can mean early dementia for some and early heart failure for others. By such studies, we may achieve our ultimate goal: to obtain the highest quality of life for all of our elderly citizens.

REFERENCES

Andrews, A.D.; S.F. Barrett; and J.I. Robbins. 1978. "Xeroderma Pigmentosum Neurological Abnormalities Correlates with Colony-Forming Ability after Ultraviolet Radiation." In *Proceedings of the National Academy of Science*, 75:1984–88.

Beckman, G. 1973. "Population Studies in Northern Sweden. VI: Polymorphism of Superoxide Dismutase." *Hereditas*, 73:305–10.

Beckman, G.; L. Beckman; and L.O. Nilsson. 1975. "Genetics of Human Superoxide Dismutase." *Hereditas*, 79: 43–46.

Bodmer, W.F.; J.R. Batchelor; J.G. Bodmer; H. Festenstein; and P.J. Morris, eds. 1978. "Histocompatibility Testing 1977." *Report of the*

Seventh International Histocompatibility Workshop and Conference. Copenhagen: Munksgaard.

Buckton, K.E.; M.L. O'Riordan; S. Ratcliffe; J. Slight; M. Mitchell; S. McBeath; A.J. Keay; D. Barr; and M. Short. 1980. "A G-Band Study of Chromosomes in Liveborn Infants." *Annals of Human Genetics* 43:227–39.

Bush, G.L.; S.M. Case; A.C. Wilson; J.L. Patton. 1977. "Rapid Speciation and Chromosomal Evolution in Mammals." *Proceedings of the National Academy of Science* 74:3942–46.

Burnet, M. 1974. *Intrinsic Mutagenesis: A Genetic Approach to Aging.* New York: Wiley.

Comfort, A. 1979. *The Biology of Senescence,* 3rd ed. New York: Elsevier.

Cutler, R.G. 1975. "Evolution of Human Longevity and the Genetic Complexity Governing Aging Rate." *Proceedings of the National Academy of Science* 72:4665–68.

Dutrillaux, B. 1975. "Sur la Nature et l'Origine des Chromosomes Humains." In *Monographes des Annales de Genetique,* pp. 1–140. Paris: Expansion Scientifique.

Evans, H.J.; R.A. Buckland; and M.L. Pardue. 1974. "Location of the Genes Coding for 18S and 28S Ribosomal RNA in the Human Genome." *Chromosoma* 48:405–26.

Feaster, W.W.; L.W. Kwok; and C.J. Epstein. 1977. "Dosage Effects for Superoxide Dismutase-1 in Nucleated Cells Aneuploid for Chromosome 21." *American Journal of Human Genetics* 29:563–70.

Finch, C.E. 1976. "Physiological Changes of Aging in Mammals." *Quarterly Review of Biology* 51:49–83.

Harris, H., and D.A. Hopkinson. 1972. "Average Heterozygosity per Locus in Man: An Estimate Based on the Incidence of Enzyme Polymorphisms." *Annals of Human Genetics* 36:9–20.

Hart, R.W., and F.B. Daniel. 1980. "Genetic Stability *in vitro* and *in vivo.*" In *Aging, Cancer and Cell Membranes,* edited by C. Borek, C.M. Fenoglin, and D.W. King, pp. 123–41. New York: Thieme-Stratton.

Hart, R.W., and R.B. Setlow. 1974. "Correlations between Deoxyribonucleic Acid Excision-Repair and Life-Span in a Number of Mammalian Species." *Proceedings of the National Academy of Science* 71:2169–73.

Jacobs, P.A. 1977. "Human Chromosomal Heteromorphisms (Variants)." *Progress in Medical Genetics* 11:251–74.

McCord, J.M., and I. Fridovich. 1968. "The Reduction of Cytochrome C by Milk Xanthine Oxidase." *Journal of Biological Chemistry* 342:5753–60.

McCord, J.M., and I. Fridovich. 1969. "Superoxide Dismutase." *Journal of Biological Chemistry* 244:6049–55.

McKusick, V. 1975. *Mendelian Inheritance in Man*, 4th edition. Baltimore: Johns Hopkins University Press.

Martin, G.M. 1978. "Genetic Syndromes in Man with Potential Relevance to the Pathobiology of Aging." In *Genetic Effects on Aging*, edited by D. Bergsma and D. Harrison. New York: A.R. Liss.

Murdoch, J.C.; J.C. Rodgers; S.S. Rao; C.D. Fletcher; and M.G. Dunningan. 1977. "Down Syndrome—Atheroma-Free Model." *British Medical Journal* 2:226–28.

Pieragostini, P.; F. Girotti; and M. Midulla. 1969. "Lipodistropia e Gigantismo en un Bambino cen Tumore Endocarnico." *Minerva Pediatrica* 21:1836–39.

Pierron, H.; H. Perrimond; and A. Orsini. 1967. "Lipoatrophie Generalisée chez un Enfant de Trois Ans par Tumeur Diencephalique." *Archives Français de Pediatrie* 24:827.

Reid, A.H., and A.F.J. Maloney. 1974. "Giant Cell Arteritis and Arateriolitis Associated with Amyloid Angiopathy in an Elderly Mongol." *Acta Neuropathologica* 27:131–37.

Robbins, J.H. 1974. "Xeroderma Pigmentosum: An Inherited Disease with Sun Sensitivity, Multiple Cutaneous Neoplasms and Abnormal DNA Repair." *Annals of Internal Medicine* 80:221–48.

Sacher, G.A. 1970. "Possible New Animals." In *Report on the Continuing Conference on the Future. II: The Age of Synthesis*, edited by M. May, pp. 23–34. Buffalo: Center for Theoretical Biology.

Sacher, G.A. 1975. "Mutation and Longevity in Relation to Cranial Capacity in Hominid Evolution." In *Antecedents of Man and After. Volume I: Primates: Functional Morphology and Evolution*, edited by R.H. Tuttle, pp. 417–42. The Hague: Mouton.

Sacher, G.A., and R.W. Hart. 1978. "Longevity, Aging and Comparative Cellular and Molecular Biology of the House Mouse, *Mus musculus*, and the White-Footed Mouse, *Peromyscus leucopus*." In *Genetic Effects on Aging*, edited by D. Bergsma and D.H. Harrison, pp. 73–98. New York: A.R. Liss.

Seip, M. 1971. "Generalized Lipodystrophy." *Ergebnisse der Inneren Medizin und Kinderheilkunde* 31:59–95.

Smith, G.F., and J.M. Berg. 1976. *Down's Anomaly*, 2d edition. New York: Churchill Livingston.

Strehler, B.L. 1980. "Selective Use and Loss of DNA During Aging." In *Aging, Cancer and Cancer Membranes*, vol. 7, edited by C. Borek, C.M. Fenoglio, and D.W. King, pp. 115–122. New York: Thieme-Stratton Inc.

Tolmasoff, J.M.; T. Ono; and R.G. Cutler. 1980. "Superoxide Dismutase: Correlation with Life-Span and Specific Metabolic Rate in

Mammalian Species." *Proceedings of the National Academy of Science* 77:2777–81.

Wilson, A.C.; T.G. White; S.S. Carlan; and L.M. Cherry. 1977. "Molecular Evolution and Cytogenetics." In *Molecular Human Cytogenetics: ICN-UCLA Symposium on Molecular and Cell Biology*, vol. 7, edited by R.S. Sparkes, D.E. Comings, and D.F. Fox, pp. 375–93. New York: Academic Press.

10 NUTRITIONAL INTERVENTION IN THE AGING PROCESS

Edward J. Masoro

Before considering nutritional intervention in the aging process, a brief overview of the biology of aging is useful as a basic orientation. This overview will focus on the well-described biological characteristics of aging, with brief mention of current thinking on the basic nature of the aging process.

A striking characteristic is the marked change that occurs in most physiological functions of mammals with increasing age. These changes were graphically summarized for humans some years ago by Nathan Shock (1962). The graph in Figure 10–1 shows, for each of the parameters measured, a loss of function with increasing age from thirty years of age on. It also shows that the rate of loss differs markedly between functions: for instance, the decline in the conduction velocity of nerve impulses is not great, while that of renal plasma flow is marked. Indeed, some parameters, such as the hemoglobin content of blood, do not change at all in healthy people with increasing age. However, it must be emphasized that the data in Figure 10–1 are from cross-sectional studies, and thus the shape of the curves defining the decline in functions may in part relate to population selection or to secular phenomena rather than solely to aging. Future research involving longitu-

Figure 10–1. Age Changes in Physiological Functions, Expressed as Percentage of Mean Value at Age Thirty Years.

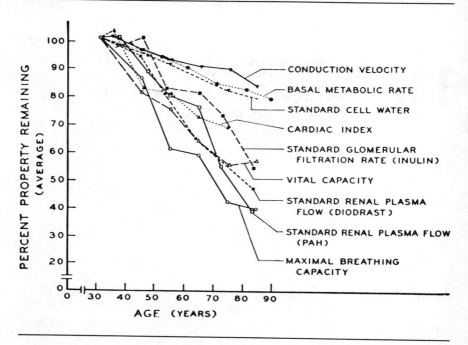

Data are derived from cross-sectional studies.
Source: Shock (1962). Reprinted with permission of the Center for the Study of Aging and Human Development, Duke University.

dinal studies of individuals is needed further to define aging effects per se.

The central issue in regard to these age-related changes in physiological functions is the effect they have on the individual. Do they lead to problems? Is one's capacity to do things reduced? Is the ability to meet biological challenges compromised? The answer to these questions is yes, as shown by the following two examples.

Dehn and Bruce (1972) analyzed data on the maximal oxygen consumption per kilogram of body weight that can be achieved by men of different ages during exercise. The maximal oxygen consumption is an index of the maximal intensity of exercise that can be sustained over an appreciable length of time. They found that between seven and eighty years of age, a continuous linear decline occurred in the maximal oxygen consumption per kilogram of body weight.

The second example is from a study carried out by Nathan Shock and his colleagues (Adler et al. 1968). They found the body fluid composition of old and young persons to be similar, but when old people were biologically challenged, they were less able to maintain body fluid composition than were young people. In one of their experiments Shock and his colleagues administered ten grams of ammonium chloride to a group of men in the third decade of life and to another group in the eighth and ninth decades. A product of ammonium chloride metabolism is hydrochloric acid. The third-decade group showed a small rise in plasma acidity, which returned to normal within eight hours. In contrast, the older group had a much greater rise in plasma acidity, which required twenty-four to seventy-two hours for its return to a normal level. This difference in response of the older group was shown to result from an age-related decline in kidney function.

The conclusion to be drawn from these studies is that with aging there is a significant loss of physiological function which results in a reduced capacity to carry out activities and a decreased ability to meet challenges. This, indeed, is a most troublesome aspect of growing old.

A second characteristic of aging is that an increased rate and probability of dying occurs after maturity has been reached (Abernethy 1979). In Figure 10–2, a set of possible survival curves for a human population is presented (Robinson 1979). The curve on the left is derived from the 1974 life expectancy compilations for American men of the U.S. Public Health Service. The shape of this curve should be contrasted with the first-order exponential decay curve (not shown in the figure) that would be obtained if death were a chance or accidental occurrence. Indeed, the survival curves of primitive human societies and unprotected animal populations are displaced toward that of an exponential decay curve. It is with the development of medical science, sanitation engineering, and other technological advances that the shape of the survival curve shown on the left was gradually attained for human populations. Since there have been no changes in the maximum length of life of human populations in recorded history

Figure 10–2. Possible Survival Curves for a Human Population.

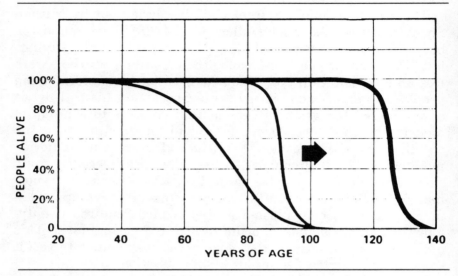

Source: Modified from Robinson (1979). Reprinted with permission from *Mechanisms of Aging and Development*.

(Robinson 1979), a reasonable projection is that the continued development of medical science and other technologies will result in survival characteristics approaching the center curve in Figure 10–2—that is, most of the population will approach the maximum length of human life. However, should aging research yield methods of extending the maximum length of human life, survival curves such as the one on the right in Figure 10–2 may be attained.

The third characteristic of aging that should be discussed is its relationship to disease. Although it has been suggested that aging is the sum total of the diseases occurring in an organism, most biologists would not feel that this is a valid concept. Loss of physiological capacity starts early in life and is progressive throughout the life span. Given a usual definition of disease, it seems unlikely that this progressive loss is secondary to disease. However, there is no question that there is a relationship between aging and disease (Upton 1977). With increasing age, there is an increased incidence of the so-called age-related or age-associated diseases, such as coronary artery disease, certain kinds of cancer, certain kinds of dementia, and so on. Moreover, a disease is likely to be more deleterious to an old person: just as ammonium chloride could not be as effectively handled by the old as by the young, so would influenza be less effectively met and more life challenging to an old person. It would seem, however, that the increased incidence of certain diseases and the increased threat of disease to life in the old are the result of the aging process, rather than disease being the cause of aging.

The general view of aging held by most biologists at this time is (1) that it involves a progressive change in one or more basic functions of either most cells or selected cells; and (2) that physiological decline, reduced ability to respond to biological challenges, and increased incidence of age-associated diseases are manifestations of a fundamental change in the functioning of protoplasm. The nature of this fundamental change is yet to be identified. Therefore, the task of biologists is twofold: one is to determine the fundamental nature of the aging process, and the other is to modulate those manifestations of aging that are now causing serious problems for individuals and for society.

FOOD RESTRICTION, LONGEVITY, AND AGING

The classic studies on food restriction and longevity were done by McCay and his colleagues (McCay, Crowell, and Maynard 1935; McCay et al. 1939). In this work, one group of weanling rats was given a balanced diet and allowed to eat ad libitum, while the second group was given the same diet but in such a restricted amount that it markedly retarded growth and development. Although many of the rats on the restricted diet died during the first year of life, those that reached one year of age lived significantly longer than the rats fed ad libitum.

Many subsequent studies on rats and other species (Barrows and Kokkonen 1977) have confirmed this life-prolonging effect of food restriction. Moreover, in the early 1960s Berg and Simms (1960, 1961) showed that levels of restriction (for instance, a 33 percent reduction in food intake) that cause little retardation in sexual maturation or in skeletal growth still significantly increase the length of life. Using a somewhat different approach, Ross (1976) further established the relationship between the amount of food intake and the length of life. In his studies, food intake was not manipulated by the experimenter; rather, the amount of food eaten by individual rats was recorded for a population of rats allowed to eat ad libitum a choice of three diets. An inverse relationship was found between how much food the rats ingested and how long they lived (Figure 10–3).

More recently, the effects of food restriction on aging have been explored in depth in our own laboratory at the University of Texas, San Antonio. Since in many respects our research has been far more extensive than previous studies, a brief description of our study seems in order. The following have been the long-term aims of this research: (1) to uncover mechanisms by which food restriction increases the length of life; (2) to analyze the aging process; and (3) to collect information for possible use in considering nutritional modification of human aging.

The design of our study is shown in Figure 10–4. Weanling (four-week-old) male specific-pathogen-free Fischer 344 male rats (n = 531) were purchased by us from the Charles River Laboratories and maintained in our barrier facility for the remainder of their lives. All the rats were fed a nutritionally complete semisynthetic diet ad libitum until six weeks of age. The rats were then divided into two groups: group A, which continued to be fed ad libitum, and group R, which was fed 60 percent of the mean ad libitum intake. Both group A and group R were subdivided into the following three subgroups: one for a longevity study, a second for the longitudinal study of body composition, and a third for cross-sectional studies of physiological and biochemical parameters.

The results of the longevity study can be summarized as follows: for the group A rats (n = 115) the mean length of life was 701± 10 days, median length of life 711 days, and maximum length of life 963 days; for the group R rats (n = 115) the mean length of life was 986 ± 25 days, the median length of life 1,046 days, and the maximum length of life 1,435 days. By plotting survival curves for group A and group R, like those for

Figure 10–3. Relationship of Quantity of Food Consumed by Male Rats Given Freedom of Dietary Choice to Length of Life.

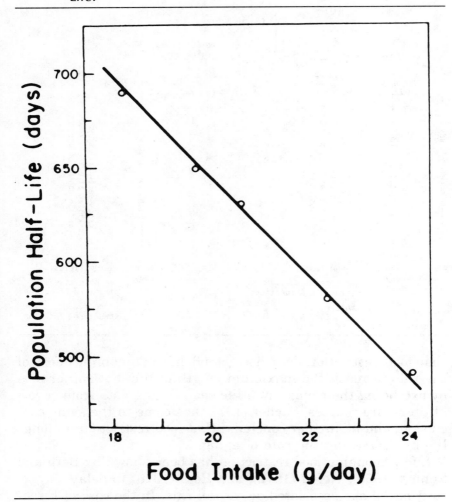

Source: Ross (1976). Reprinted with permission.

humans depicted in Figure 10–2, one sees that food restriction had two effects: first, it shifted the entire curve to the right; and second, the slope of the curve for group R rats between the 90 percent and 10 percent survival points was much less steep than the slope of the curve for group A rats. These facts show

Figure 10–4.   Design of Food-Restriction Study

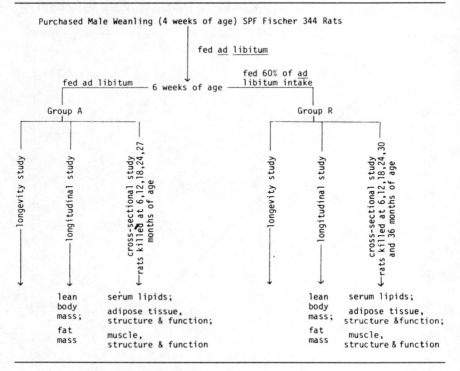

that food restriction does not extend life by enabling most of the rats to reach the maximum length of life, but rather acts by extending their maximum life span. Using data from several literature sources, Sacher (1977) has come to the same conclusion, and he further concludes that food restriction prolongs life by decreasing the rate of aging.

Life-prolonging food restriction has been shown by Berg and Simms (1960), Nolen (1972), and Ross (1976) to delay the occurrence of age-associated disease in rats. In the case of Fischer 344 male rats, the strain used in our study, one research group (Coleman et al. 1977) reported that these rats have two major age-associated lesions, testicular interstitial cell tumors and chronic nephropathy. They classified the latter by five grades, grades 1, 2, 3, 4, and end stage, in order of increasing severity. In our study, neither group A nor group R rats showed any evidence of chronic nephropathy until eighteen months of age, when all of the rats sacrificed from both groups had either grade 1 or 2 lesions. By twenty-four months of age, more than 80 percent of the sacrificed group A rats had grade 3 lesions, while grade 3 lesions were not observed at all in group R rats until thirty months of age and occurred in less than 35 percent of the group R rats sacrificed at thirty-six months of age. With regard to testicular interstitial cell tumors, food restriction was found to delay their appearance; almost all of the group A rats had the tumors by eighteen months of age, whereas group R rats did not show these tumors until thirty months of age.

Most of the group A rats died between eighteen and thirty months of age. On the basis of end-stage nephropathy lesions and clinical findings, renal failure was the probable cause of death of more than 90 percent of these rats. Most of the group R rats died between thirty and forty-two months of age, and there were three major probable causes of death: renal failure, vascular rupture, and hepatic degeneration, each accounting for about 30 percent of the deaths. It thus appears that life-prolonging food restriction does not alter the age of the first appearance of chronic nephropathy, but markedly delays its rate of progression from grade 1 to end stage. It is not clear whether death from vascular rupture and hepatic degeneration in the group R rats is a direct result of the restricted diet or simply relates to the long length of life of these rats; for example, group A rats might also have died from these causes had their life span been longer.

While many factors have been suggested as responsible for the life-prolonging action of food restriction (Young 1979), the following have received serious consideration: (1) prolonged immaturity; (2) reduced rate and prolonged duration of growth; (3) reduction in fat or adipose tissue; and (4) caloric restriction and its metabolic consequences. It seems worthwhile, therefore, to briefly consider the information currently available in regard to these hypotheses.

McCay, Crowler, and Maynard (1935) and McCay et al. (1939) based their classic studies on the hypothesis that prolonged immaturity would result in the extension of the life span, and they felt their findings strongly supported this view. However, Berg and Simms (1961, 1969) found that less severe food restriction, causing little retardation of development, also prolonged life. Moreover, Stuchlikova, Juricova-Horokova, and Deyl (1975) showed that food restriction is effective in prolonging life in rats even when started as late as the end of the first year of life, which is well past the developmental phase. It therefore seems that prolonged immaturity is probably not importantly involved in the life-prolonging action of food restriction.

In a rat study by Ross, Lustbader, and Bras (1975) and in a mouse study by Goodrick (1977), growth rate correlated negatively and duration of growth correlated positively with length of life, but maximum attained weight did not correlate with length of life. In contrast, in a study of rats by Everitt and Webb (1957), duration of growth correlated positively and maximum size attained correlated negatively with length of life, but no correlation was seen with rate of growth. In our study, data were collected on the changes with age in both body weight and lean body mass in the group A and group R rats. Group A rats grew faster and reached a higher maximum body weight than group R rats (mean maximum body weight for group A was 545 grams; for group R, 300 grams). Group A rats attained a significantly greater maximal lean body mass than Group R rats. In both group A and group R rats, lean body mass reached its maximum value at about 60 percent of the life span, after which it changed little until just before death, when in most cases it fell markedly. This work confirmed an earlier report by Lesser, Deutsch, and Markofsky (1973).

Thus it is seen that, unlike the human, the rat does not show a continuous fall in lean body mass during adult life. Although group R rats have a slower growth rate, longer duration of growth, lower body weight, and smaller lean body mass than group A rats, these findings do not establish whether all or any of these factors are responsible for the longer length of life of group R rats. Since within the group A rat population, there was a broad spectrum of growth rates and maximum weights attained, analyses of these data were carried out to seek information on the possible causal role of these factors.

The growth of the group A rats during the first year or so of life fits an exponential growth model quite well. Analyses based on this model showed that the growth rate at four months of age (a time of rapid growth) is negatively correlated with length of life (n = 114, $r = -0.34, p < 0.001$) and that the maximal exponential weight is also negatively correlated with length of life (n = 114, $r = -0.21, p < 0.05$). No correlation was found between duration of exponential growth and length of life. Reduction in growth rates may therefore be a factor in the life-prolonging action of food restriction.

A widely proposed and popular thesis holds that a reduction in fat mass or adipose tissue mass has a life-prolonging action (Young 1979). In this regard, adipose tissue was studied by our group throughout the life span of group A and group R rats. Total fat mass was found to increase during adult life in both group A and group R rats until about 70 percent of the life span, after which it declined with advancing age. Results from the longitudinal study on group A rats (Bertrand, Lynd, Masoro, and Yu 1980), are shown in Figure 10–5. Group R rats were found to have a smaller total adipose mass than group A rats. The results of the cross-sectional study on the epididymal and perirenal fat depots are in agreement with these findings. In group A rats, both depots reached maximum mass at eighteen months of age and declined at more advanced ages (Figure 10–6), while in group R rats the depots reached maximum mass at thirty months of age and again declined at more advanced ages. At all ages studied in common, the depots of group R rats were smaller than those of group A rats. Changes in the mass of a fat depot result from either a change in volume of the fat cells (adipocytes) making up a depot or a change in the number of fat cells in the depot or both. Figures 10–7 and 10–8 show that the increase in adipose mass through middle age in group A rats involved both an increase in fat cell volume and fat cell number. Indeed, the perirenal depot of group A rats grew almost entirely by increasing the number of adipocytes, a surprising finding since it has been generally believed that fat cell number is fixed in adults. The loss of depot mass during senescence was almost totally due to a reduction in the volume of the fat cells, with no significant change seen in number of cells.

Figure 10–5. Fat Mass Changes during the Life Span of Six of the Group A Rats of a Longitudinal Study of Total Fat Mass

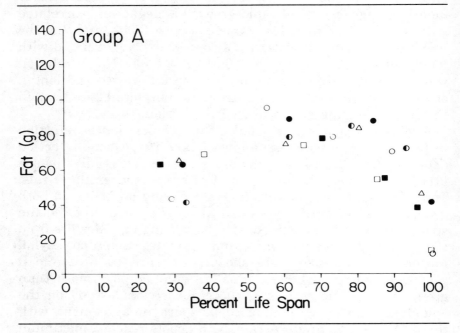

Note: Each of the symbols on the graph refers to a different rat.

Source: Bertrand, (1980). Reprinted with permission from the *Journal of Gerontology*.

The lower fat mass in group R rats does not appear to be a factor in the life-prolonging action of food restriction. This conclusion is based on the following analysis: In the group A rat population, there is no significant correlation between length of life and percent body fat at eight months of age or maximum measured absolute fat mass or maximum measured absolute percent body fat. Moreover, in the group R rat population, there is no significant correlation between length of life and percentage body fat at eight months of age, but there is a significant positive correlation between length of life and maximum measured absolute fat mass or maximum measured percentage body fat ($r = 0.63$, $p < 0.001$).

That caloric restriction and its metabolic consequences are a factor in the life-prolonging action of food restriction has yet to be unequivocally demonstrated. On the one hand, there are two lines of evidence to support this hypothesis. First, Ross and Bras (1973) have shown that in rats fed diets widely differing in composition, restriction of the amount eaten (i.e., the caloric intake) in each instance increased the length of life. Second, on the basis of data of Ross (1969), Sacher (1977) points out that when caloric intake is expressed as kilocalories

Figure 10–6.   Changes with Age in the Mass of the Epididymal and Perirenal Depots

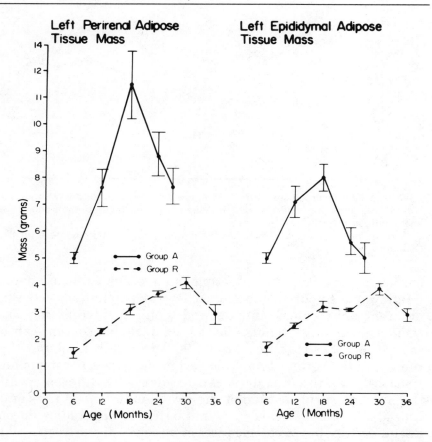

Note: Values recorded are means ± SEM, the n = 10 except for twenty-seven-month-old group A rats where n = 9. The solid lines refer to group A rats and the broken lines to group R rats.

Source: Bertrand et al. (1980). Reprinted with permission from the *Journal of Gerontology*.

Figure 10–7. Changes with Age in the Mean Volume of the Adipocyte Population in the Epididymal and Perirenal Depots

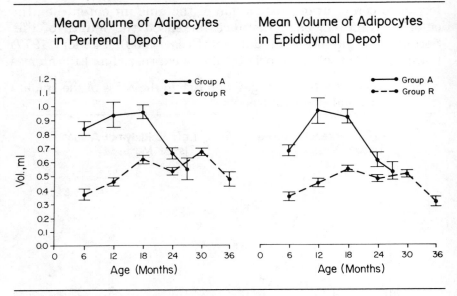

Mean Volume of Adipocytes in Perirenal Depot   Mean Volume of Adipocytes in Epididymal Depot

Note: Values recorded are means ± SEM, the n = 10 except for the twenty-seven-month-old group A rats where n = 9. The solid lines refer to group A rats and broken lines to group R rats.

Source: Bertrand et al. (1980). Reprinted with permission from the *Journal of Gerontology*.

per gram body weight per lifetime, an average value of approximately one hundred is obtained for rat populations fed very different daily caloric intakes and diets of different compositions. On the other hand, evidence against this concept can be seen in another study by Ross (1969) in which he found that the average lifetime total caloric intake between rat populations fed two different diets can be markedly different, while the average survival time of the two populations is the same. Indeed, Ross (1976) clearly points out that his studies do not unequivocally prove caloric restriction is the factor responsible for the life-prolonging action of food restriction.

It is clear that none of the suggestions thus far proposed has provided a fruitful approach to the experimental exploration of the mechanisms involved in the life-prolonging action of food restriction. In 1970, when we first became interested in this phenomenon, we were surprised to learn that little work had been done on the effect of food restriction on the biochemical and physiological changes that occur with age. It was our belief that exploration of the effects of food restriction on these age-related functional changes might well provide clues to the mechanisms underlying the life-prolonging action. It was for this reason that we have focused much of our research effort

Figure 10–8. Changes with Age in the Number of Adipocytes in the Epididymal and Perirenal Depots

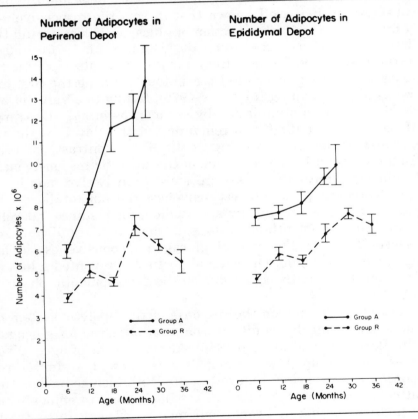

Note: Values recorded are means ± SEM, the n = 10 except for twenty-seven-month-old group A rats where n = 9. The solid lines refer to group A rats and the broken lines to group R rats.

Source: Bertrand et al. (1980). Reprinted with permission from the *Journal of Gerontology*.

on exploring the effects of food restriction on selected aspects of age-related biochemical and physiological changes. Others also have had this line of thought. For instance, Walford and his colleagues (Walford et al. 1974; Weindruch et al. 1979) and Fernandes and his colleagues (1976, 1978) recently showed that the age-related deterioration of the immune system is delayed by food restriction.

Of the functions we have studied, the effect of hormones on isolated fat cell lipolysis is perhaps the most interesting. The rate of lipolysis in isolated fat cells is an index of the rate of fat mobilization, a process regulated by hormones and the nervous system. It is well known that in rats the responsiveness of fat cells to the lipolytic action of glucagon is lost during the first few weeks of postweaning life (Holm et al. 1976). Indeed in the case of the fat cells from our group A rats, lipolytic responsiveness to glucagon fell precipitously during the first few weeks of postweaning life (Voss 1979), falling to a value of approximately zero stimulation by six months of age (Bertrand, Masoro, and Yu 1980) and remaining at that level for the remainder of the life span (Figure 10–9). In contrast, fat cells from our group R rats lost none of the lipolytic responsiveness to glucagon until the rats were more than twelve months of age. Moreover, glucagon responsiveness did not totally disappear in group R rats at any age studied; for instance, fat cells from thirty-six-month-old rats still showed a significant response. Thus, in the case of glucagon responsiveness of fat cells, food restriction delayed and partially prevented a loss in function that usually occurs during the developmental phase of life.

The effects of age on the response of the lipolytic system of fat cells to epinephrine differs from that observed for glucagon (Yu, Bertrand, and Masoro 1980). At six months of age, adipocytes from group A and group R rats showed a similar response to epinephrine (Figure 10–10). With increasing age, the fat cells from group A rats lost responsiveness to epinephrine (a nadir occurring at twenty-four months of age). In contrast, there was no loss in responsiveness to epinephrine in adipocytes from group R rats until after eighteen months of age, and the extent of loss was much less marked than in group A rats even when group R rats reached very old age (up to thirty-six

Figure 10–9. Effects of Age on the Response of Isolated Adipocytes to the Lipolytic Action of Glucagon (1 microgram).

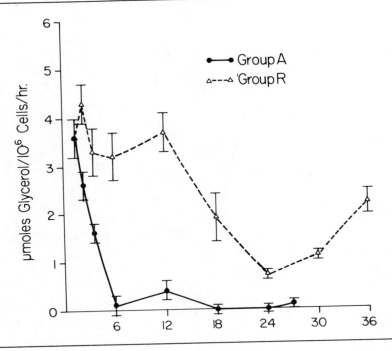

Note: Data are expressed as micromoles glycerol released above the basal rate/10⁶ cells/hour. The values are means for ten or more rats except for the twenty-seven-month-old group A rats where the n = 9.

Source: Derived from the studies of Bertrand, Masoro, and Yu (1980) and of Voss (1979). Reprinted with permission from the *Journal of Gerontology*.

months). Again we see that food restriction delays an age-related loss in function, but in this case it is a loss that starts after maturity has been reached rather than in the developmental stage of life.

Are these studies with isolated fat cells indicative of changes in the fat mobilization system of the intact rat? On the basis of studies (Liepa et al. 1980) of the postabsorptive serum free fatty acid (FFA) levels in group A and group R (Figure 10–11), the answer appears to be yes. Serum FFA levels are a good index of the rate of fat mobilization. At six months of age the postabsorptive FFA levels of group A and group R rats are

Figure 10–10. Effects of Age on the Lipolytic Response of Epididymal Adipocytes to 10^{-5}M Epinephrine

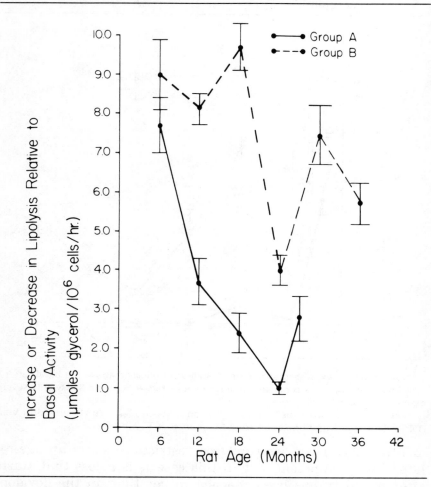

Note: Data are expressed as micromoles glycerol released above the basal rate/10^6cells/hour. For the group A rats, the values are means ± standard errors for ten, ten, ten, ten, and nine rats at six, twelve, eighteen, twenty-four, and twenty-seven months of age, respectively. For the group R rats, the values are means ± standard errors for ten, ten, ten, seven, ten, and ten rats at six, twelve, eighteen, twenty-four, thirty, and thirty-six months of age, respectively.

Source: Yu et al. (1980). Reproduced with permission from *Metabolism* 29, no. 5 (May 1980): 438-44.

Figure 10–11. Age and the Postabsorptive Serum FFA Levels of Group A and Group R Rats

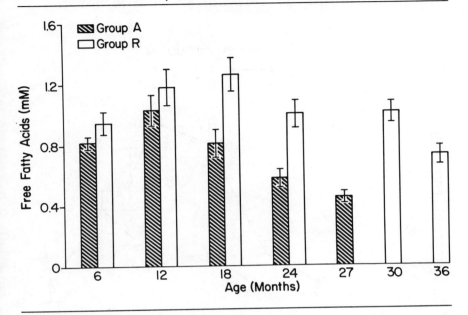

Note: For group A rats, the values are means ± standard errors for ten, nine, ten, ten, and ten rats at six, twelve, eighteen, twenty-four and twenty-seven months of age, respectively. For the group R rats, the values are means ± standard errors for ten, ten, nine, ten, eight, and ten rats at six, twelve, eighteen, twenty-four, thirty, and thirty-six months of age, respectively.

Source: Liepa et al. (1980). Reproduced with permission from the *American Journal of Physiology*.

similar. With increasing age the postabsorptive FFA levels fall in the group A rats, but in the group R rats this fall is delayed and much less marked.

This modulation of age-related physiological change is not restricted to fat mobilization, as shown in Figure 10–12 where the age-related changes in serum cholesterol (Liepa et al. 1980) in group A and group R rats are presented. At six months of age, group A and group R rats have similar serum cholesterol levels. With increasing age, group A rats show a marked increase in serum cholesterol levels. However, it is not until thirty months of age that the serum cholesterol level in

Figure 10–12. Age and the Postabsorptive Serum Total Cholesterol Levels of Group A and Group R Rats

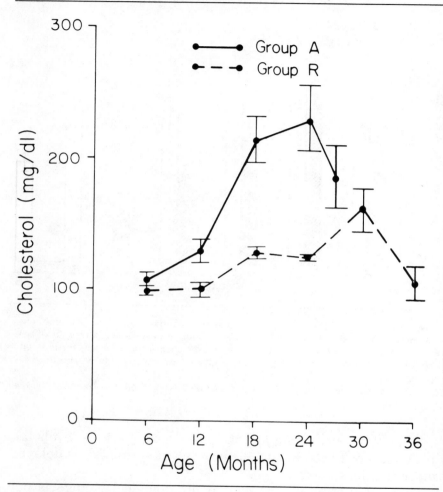

Note: For the group A rats, the values are means ± standard errors for nine, seven, ten, ten, and nine rats at six, twelve, eighteen, twenty-four, and twenty-seven months of age, respectively. For the group R rats, the values are means ± standard errors for six, nine, ten, ten, ten, and ten rats at six, twelve, eighteen, twenty-four, thirty, and thirty-six months of age, respectively.

Source: Liepa et al. (1980). Reproduced with permission from the *American Journal of Physiology*.

group R rats is in the same range as that exhibited by group A rats at eighteen months of age.

The foregoing experiments together with others from our study, as well as those of Walford and colleagues and Fernandes and colleagues, clearly indicate that age-related changes in the physiological and biochemical systems are markedly delayed by food restriction. They thus provide a starting point for analyzing the mechanisms by which food restriction acts to prolong life.

In my opinion, future research should be focused on the following four areas:

1. The possible role of a specific dietary factor or factors in the action of food restriction requires further research. Studies on the role of proteins, carbohydrates, and fats have been done, but the results have not been convincing. Although research in this area is both costly and difficult to execute definitively, answers to these questions have such great potential in terms of the modulation of human aging that it should be a high-priority research area.

2. A second important area of study is concerned with the period of the life span and the duration of the life span required for food restriction to effect its modulating influence on aging. Not only is this information of theoretical interest, but it is also immensely important in the practical context of possibly modulating human aging by nutritional means.

3. There is obviously a great need to learn whether the life-prolonging action of food restriction relates only to laboratory rodents or to other mammals as well. However, the resources needed to carry out such a study are almost prohibitive. Rats, mice, and most other laboratory rodents have a sufficiently short life span to permit an analysis of life-prolonging procedures within four to five years. This length of time is feasible within the constraints of both the working life of the researcher and the granting systems of most funding agencies. It is difficult to envision funding and executing such work on cats or dogs or nonhuman primates. One hope is that if future work establishes that

food restriction is effective when carried out during only a part of the adult life of rodents, it may be possible to study longer lived species within a manageable time framework.

4. Research on the molecular mechanisms by which food restriction influences aging is of great importance because it may provide basic information about the aging process. For example, we have recently found that food restriction prevents the age-related loss in responsiveness of adipocytes to the lipolytic action of glucagon, either by influencing the glucagon receptor in the plasma membrane of the fat cell or by affecting the transduction of the signal between the receptor and the adenylate cyclase system of that cell. Indeed, when explored at a molecular level, the modulating influence of food restriction on age-related physiological changes may add much to our understanding of the aging process.

REFERENCES

Abernethy, J.D. 1979. "The Exponential Increase in Mortality Rate with Age Attributed to Wearing-Out of Biological Components." *Journal of Theoretical Biology* 80:333–54.

Adler, S.; R.D. Lindeman; M.J. Yiengst; E. Beard; and N.W. Shock. 1968. "Effect of Acute Acid Loading on Urinary Acid Excretion by the Aging Human Kidney." *Journal of Laboratory and Clinical Medicine* 72:278–89.

Barrows, C.H., and G.C. Kokkonen. 1977. "Relationship between Nutrition and Aging." In *Advances in Nutritional Research*, Vol. I, edited by Harold H. Draper, pp. 253–98. New York: Plenum Publishing Corporation.

Berg, B.N., and H.S. Simms. 1960. "Nutrition and Longevity. II: Longevity and the Onset of Disease with Different Levels of Food Intake." *Journal of Nutrition* 71:255–63.

Berg, B.N., and H.S. Simms. 1961. "Nutrition and Longevity. III: Food Restriction beyond 800 Days." *Journal of Nutrition* 74:23–32.

Bertrand, H.A.; F.T. Lynd; E.J. Masoro; and B.P. Yu. 1980. "Changes in Adipose Mass and Cellularity through the Adult Life of Rats Fed Ad Libitum or a Life-Prolonging Restricted Diet." *Journal of Gerontology* 36:827–35.

Bertrand, H.A.; E.J. Masoro; and B.P. Yu. 1980. "Maintenance of Glucagon Promoted Lipolysis in Adipocytes by Food Restriction." *Endocrinology* 107:591–95.

Coleman, G.L.; S.W. Barthold; G.W. Osbaldiston; S.J. Foster; and A.M. Jonas. 1977. "Pathological Changes during Aging in Barrier-Reared Fischer 344 Male Rats." *Journal of Gerontology* 32:258–78.

Dehn, M.M., and R.A. Bruce. 1972. "Longitudinal Variations in Maximal Oxygen Intake with Age and Activity." *Journal of Applied Physiology* 33:805–07.

Everitt, A.V., and C. Webb. 1957. "The Relation between Body Weight Changes and Life Duration in Male Rats." *Journal of Gerontology* 12:128–35.

Fernandes, G.; P. Friend; E.J. Yunis; and R.A. Good. 1978. "Influence of Dietary Restriction on Immunologic Function and Renal Disease in (NXBXNAW)F$_1$ Mice." In *Proceedings of the National Academy of Science* 75:1500–04.

Fernandes, , G.; E.J. Yunis; and R.A. Good. 1976. "Influence of Diet on Survival of Mice." In *Proceedings of the National Academy of Science* 73:1279–83.

Goodrick, C.L. 1977. "Body Weight Change over the Life Span and Longevity for 657 BL/6J Mice and Mutations which Differ in Maximal Body Weight." *Gerontology* 23:405–13.

Holm, G.; B. Jacobson; P. Bjorntorp; and U. Smith. 1976. "Effects of Age and Cell Size on Rat Adipose Metabolism." *Journal of Lipid Research* 16:461–64.

Lesser, G.T.; S. Deutsch; and J. Markofsky. 1973. "Aging in the Rat: Longitudinal and Cross-Sectional Studies of Body Composition." *American Journal of Physiology* 225:1472–78.

Liepa, G.U.; E.J. Masoro; H.A. Bertrand; and B.P. Yu. 1980. "Food Restriction as a Modulator of Age-Related Changes in Serum Lipid." *American Journal of Physiology* 238:E253–E257.

McCay, C.M.; M.F. Crowell; and L.A. Maynard. 1935. "The Effect of Retarded Growth upon the Length of Life Span and upon the Ultimate Body Size." *Journal of Nutrition* 10:63–79.

McCay, C.M.; L.A. Maynard; G. Sperling; and L. Barnes. 1939. "Retarded Growth, Life Span, Ultimate Body Size and Age Changes in the Albino Rat after Feeding Diets Restricted in Calories." *Journal of Nutrition* 18:1–13.

Nolen, G.A. 1972. "Effect of Various Restricted Dietary Regimens on the Growth, Health and Longevity of Albino Rats." *Journal of Nutrition* 102:1477–94.

Robinson, A.B. 1979. "Molecular Clocks, Molecular Profiles and Optimum Diets; Three Approaches to the Problem of Aging." *Mechanisms of Aging and Development* 9:225–36.

Ross, M.H. 1969. "Aging, Nutrition and Hepatic Enzyme Activity Patterns in the Rat." *Journal of Nutrition* 97:565–601.

Ross, M.H. 1976. "Nutrition and Longevity in Experimental Animals." In *Nutrition and Aging*, edited by M. Winick, pp. 43–57. New York: Wiley.

Ross, M.H., and G. Bras. 1973. "Influence of Protein Under- and Over-Nutrition on Spontaneous Tumor Prevalence in the Rat." *Journal of Nutrition* 103:944–63.

Ross, M.H.; E. Lustbader; and G. Bras. 1976. "Dietary Practices and Growth Responses as Predictors of Longevity." *Nature* 262:548–53.

Sacher, G.A. 1977. "Life Table Modification and Life Prolongation." In *Handbook of the Biology of Aging*, edited by. C.E. Finch and L. Hayflick, pp. 582–638. New York: Van Nostrand Reinhold Co.

Shock, N.W. 1962. "The Science of Gerontology." In *Proceedings Seminars of the Council on Gerontology, 1959-61*. Durham: Duke University Press.

Stuchlikova, E.; M. Juricova-Horokova; and Z. Deyl. 1975. "New Aspects of the Dietary Effects of Life Prolongation in Rodents: What Is the Role of Obesity in Aging?" *Experimental Gerontology* 10:141–44.

Upton, A.C. 1977. "Pathobiology." In *Handbook of the Biology of Aging*, edited by. C.E. Finch and L. Hayflick, pp. 513–35. New York: Van Nostrand Reinhold Co.

Voss, K.H. 1979. "An Analysis of the Age-Related Loss of Glucagon-Stimulated Lipolysis." Ph.D. dissertation, University of Texas Health Science Center, San Antonio.

Walford, R.L.; R.K. Kiu; M. Delima-Berbasse; M. Mathis; and G.S. Smith. 1974. "Long-Term Dietary Restriction and Immune Function in Mice: Response to Sheep Red Blood Cells and to Mitogenic Agents." *Mechanisms of Aging and Development* 2:447–54.

Weindruch, R.H.; J.A. Kristie; K.E. Cheney; and R.L. Walford. 1979. "Influence of Controlled Dietary Restriction on Immunologic Function and Aging." *Federation Proceedings* 38:2007–16.

Young, V.R. 1979. "Diet as a Modulator of Aging and Longevity." *Federation Proceedings* 38:1994–2000.

Yu, B.P.; H.A. Bertrand; and E.J. Masoro. 1980. "Nutrition-Aging Influences of Catecholamine-Promoted Lipolysis." *Metabolism* 24:438–44.

11 MORAL ISSUES IN THE NEW QUEST FOR LONGEVITY

John B. Orr

The Homeric *Hymn to Aphrodite*, written during the seventh or eighth century B.C., contains a haunting story about the human quest for longevity. It describes the romance of Tithonus, a Trojan, and Eos, who was a daughter of the immortal Titans—a woman so beautiful and youthful that people believed her to be the personification of dawn. Because she could not bear the thought of her romance coming to an end, Eos approached one of the gods and begged him to grant Tithonus the gift of immortality. To her astonishment, her wish was granted. But in the process, Eos committed a terrible mistake: she forgot to ask that Tithonus be allowed to retain his youthfulness.

For a while, Tithonus and Eos lived happily together, luxuriating in the knowledge that Tithonus would never die. But then the truth revealed itself. Tithonus's hair turned white, and with a deadly inevitability, all the infirmities of old age fell upon him, until he could no longer lift his arms and legs. Eos had no choice but to lock her immortal lover in a dark room, where he lies eternally, babbling unintelligibly.

The unknown author of this story was admittedly not much of a philosopher. Reflecting on Tithonus's sad fate, he implied that the flowering of romance is not a good enough reason for

213

the gods to grant immortality. Romance, after all, is a passing fancy. The author's more profound point, however, is that it is unnatural for mortals to escape death: only the gods should be immortal.

The story of Tithonus can be read in other ways, and with little fear of retaliation by the ancient author, I will develop my own, modern-day commentary, based on the assumption that Eos's quest to secure longevity for her lover continues still, perhaps in an even more obsessive fashion. Today Eos is a pharmaceutical corporation employee, experimenting with possibilities for arresting cellular breakdown and therefore, for extending life. Or she is a nutritionist, looking for clues as to how alterations in a person's diet can raise the chances for a longer life. Or she is a researcher, beseeching gods at the National Institutes of Health to bestow funds that may finally result in weapons to attack death-dealing diseases.

Tithonus also has his contemporary counterparts. He is someone who is enchanted with life and who does not want to give it up. He jogs, frequents the local health club, adheres to the latest diet, takes vitamin C, and tries to repress the personality traits that he thinks will induce heart attacks. In short, Tithonus is the one who wants a little more romance with the delights of this world, and who turns to various and assorted Eoses for help in making that romance possible.

Human beings apparently cannot give up their thirst for greater longevity. But they do not want to share Tithonus's fate either. Like the Hesiodic hymn, our current thinking on longevity conveys both an affirmation and a warning—an affirmation that such a quest for longevity is an obvious good, but a warning that the quest involves dangers and complex moral issues which are too easily overlooked.

THE RIGHT TO LIFE

From one perspective, Tithonus and Eos probably got what they deserved. Tithonus was mortal, not a god. And it was presumptuous on the part of the couple to think that a mortal should be able to escape from the limits of his creatureliness. By accepting immortality, Tithonus committed the sin of pride.

He was rightly punished, and in the best way possible: by having to suffer in a limitless way the pains of mortality—an aching back, senility, stiff joints, hurting feet. Within both the Greco-Roman and the Jewish-Christian traditions that have shaped our culture's values, it has always been viewed as a tragedy when people try to be godlike. The effort always ends in failure.

Within these traditions, though, it has never been viewed as a sin merely to desire a long life. Long life is perceived as a reward for virtue, as a special gift. Indeed, many Biblical scholars believe that one of the major ideas of the Jewish and Christian scriptures, often overlooked, is the assertion that God created people with the possibility of life without death. According to the mythographer James Frazer (1918), for example, the earliest forms of the story of Adam and Eve suggested the possibility of extended longevity. The two trees in Eden were the tree of life and the tree of death, Frazer suggests. God told Adam and Eve to eat from the tree of life, but a serpent tricked them into eating from the tree of death. Thus people were not made to die. They were tricked into death—they brought death on themselves.

Strange as this idea may seem, it is consistently present even in the later Christian scriptures. Death came into the world because of sin, the New Testament writer Paul declared. He spoke about the Old Adam, and by this he meant all people from the beginning of time who in one way or another had chosen death because of the refusal to live in obedience to their creator. Naturally enough, then, when a newly converted Christian, Paul discussed the possibility of a New Adam—a people who would no longer be rebellious against their God—he had to consider the possibility that human life could once again be freed from the awful specter of death.

Contrary to popular impression, Paul never said that by giving allegiance to the new messiah Jesus people would be given *immortality of the soul.* Jesus was not viewed by Paul as a reincarnation of Eos, capable of inducing the Creator to infuse a quality or a substance into believers' souls that would provide insurance against death. Rather, Paul spoke more radically about a "resurrection of the body" (see especially 1 Corinthians 15). The idea implied a promise that Christians could and would participate in Jesus' own resurrection, and that their deathless life would not be as an ephemeral, amorphous soul. Eternal life was pictured as a resurrection of a person's recognizable self, body and all (albeit in a "transformed" state).

Much of the value of looking back at these early myths and scriptures lies in recognizing that Western people have been influenced by them, whether or not they currently think of themselves as religious. Deep, deep in our cultural heritage is the Greek, Jewish, and Christian belief that life is good, that death is bad, and that death is to be overcome. This belief is almost commonsense for us. We cannot imagine affirming the opposite. Occasionally, of course, a person like Schopenhauer argues the case for suicide, and serious thinkers formulate reasons why people have a right to die if pain and hopelessness turn death into a state to be preferred. But hardly anyone wants to transform these arguments about the right to die into a general philosophy. In Western culture we think about life in a moralistic way. It is good to be living. Life is a value to be affirmed.

A corollary in Western culture is that a longer life is better than a shorter one. This is not an absolute conviction, however. As Tithonus discovered, long life sometimes brings pain and disintegration. So the life we value becomes progressively mixed with death, until the final experience of death may come as a welcome relief, as a friend, as a natural stage in life, as a "death in good time," or even as a joyous event.

But even when death is viewed as an approaching friend, by far the dominant passion in Western culture is to fight that friend and thereby demonstrate our commitment to the preservation and prolongation of life. This passion is notably present in the various oaths and codes that spell out the obligations of the medical profession. Although the Hippocratic Corpus, for example, did allow physicians in extreme cases "to refuse to treat those who are overmastered by their diseases, realizing that in such cases medicine is powerless," the physician's task was clearly specified by the obligation to treat the sick, to lessen "the violence of disease," and to fend off the approaching death. Thomas Percival's nineteenth century code of medical ethics heightened that obligation. Percival argued that physicians should not let even what he called "parsimonious considerations"—that is, issues related to potential financial burdens—stand in the way of "prescribing wine, and drugs even of high price, when required in diseases of extraordinary malignity and danger." So defined, the medical profession simply assumes that death is the enemy. The assumption is not debated. Life, where it exists, as long as it is "human," should be prolonged.

This obligation to protect and extend life is especially clear in the public debate about abortion. The discussion about the rights of women to decide responsibility concerning their desire to bear children, for example, is limited by the shared conviction that living human fetuses must be protected. The abortion issue finally becomes an argument about criteria for determining exactly at what point a fetus must be regarded as a living human being. Human beings have a right to life. There is no question about that—only about who is a human being.

The extent to which the medical profession is committed to the prolongation of life seems somehow best dramatized by the precision required in defining life when support systems are withdrawn from terminally ill patients. There is little room here for loose generalizing—for imaging human life in terms of what people might view as the "truly" human, the fully functioning, potentially self-realizing individual. The life to be prolonged includes life at the lowest possible level where it is still appropriate to speak about the presence of the "human." Some argue, for example, that human life is present and subject to protection when there is a simple capacity to breathe without life-support systems. Others argue that life must be indicated by the presence of certain higher brain functions. However the issue is defined, impressive barriers exist against forcing physicians to judge which lives are sufficiently worthy of protection. The commitment to life itself, at its lowest level, is very, very deep in our culture.

Thus, in the climate created by Jewish-Christian and Greco-Roman values, we can claim for ourselves a natural right to life. At the very least, this is experienced as a right not to be murdered—not to have one's life terminated by someone else for reasons other than (perhaps) war or (perhaps) self-defense. The right to life, however, implies something more. It implies the right to longevity and seems even to suggest the positive obligation of a society to provide for "health"—that is, to provide conditions that will maximize the chances of individuals to live as long as possible. Our right to life involves, at least by implication, as much taste of immortality as an individual's luck, wisdom, and medical technology can provide.

Therefore, in terms of the story of Tithonus, Eos may have been unjustly punished. She was merely exercising her right to secure as much life as possible for her love. If she lapsed into the sin of pride, that was indeed a punishable crime. But the gods themselves were perhaps in error in confusing Eos's desire for Tithonus's immortality with a supposed desire to make Tithonus into a god. After all, in nearby Palestine, the God of the Jews had already learned through the story of Adam and Eve that the desire for immortality and the prideful rebellion against God were two different things. The God of the Jews knew that it was only human to want as much life as possible, and in Palestine it was viewed as a tragedy that human sin had denied people an immortality that had once been theirs.

But what kind of right is this right to a prolonged life? It is surely an unusual one, if only because rights always involve obligations on someone's part. If I have a right to vote, for example, someone is obligated to maintain an electoral system to which I have regular, assured access. If I legitimately can claim a right to private property, someone has an obligation to organize a legal system that determines how property can be acquired, that guarantees I can acquire property under certain conditions, and that protects me from the unfair seizure of that property. If I claim a right to prolonged life, however, who is obligated to do anything?

It does not make sense, for example, to argue that a right has been violated when a person is stricken with cancer, or when a child is run down by an automobile. These are tragedies, but they are not occasions when an injustice has occurred. Likewise, the right to prolonged life has not been violated because a local hospital has been unable to afford a particular diagnostic machine, or because governmental funds have not been amply allocated for the speedy development of drugs that will inhibit the aging process. These may be tough breaks, but not violations of rights.

My intuition is that the right to a prolonged life is best understood in the framework of something like a free-market model. People have a right to seek the longest life possible for themselves and their loved ones within a social system where reasonable opportunities to enhance the possibility for long life have been provided and where these opportunities have been fairly allocated within the population. The right to a prolonged life assumes that human longevity is on the public agenda and that it is reasonable to speak about public obligations for support of life-giving research and services.

The right to a prolonged life is experienced first, however, not as a public guarantee, but as a social acceptance of individuals' efforts to extend their own lives. People have a right to seek the longest possible life, just as people have a right to seek property, wealth, and intangibles like self-respect. Likewise, they can and often do choose to ignore the whole matter. Virtually everything from cigarettes to liquor, barbequed steaks to diet drinks, walking down stairs to swimming in the ocean have been deemed at one time or another to constitute serious dangers to life and limb. A life-style that is obsessed with winning bodily immortality is a dull life-style, perhaps even a psychically destructive one. Nevertheless, the reasonable search for a long life is neither obviously immoral nor trivial. It is one among many worthy pursuits that motivate people in the free market of human activities.

The right to a prolonged life is experienced also as a concern on the public agenda, because the private pursuit of long life by an individual can never be a wholly isolated project, independent from the network of public policies and institutions. An individual, for example, may choose to watch his or her diet and may try to eat only life-prolonging foods. And that individual may join a health maintenance program, and may regularly elect extensive physical examinations. These life-style choices will express the individual's unique pattern of preferences, but they also will presuppose a social system of opportunities for the enhancement of longevity. They will presuppose a history of government and foundation funding for research related to diet. They will depend on the availability of health institutions whose services can be purchased at a reasonable cost. And they will require the education-nurtured ability to recognize the connection between diet and longevity and between preventive medicine and the opportunity to postpone catastrophic illness.

In other words, as observed by Adam Smith, the eighteenth century defender of the free market, the individual's attempts to satisfy private goals require certain services that are not of the individual's own making. The eighteenth century entrepreneur, for example, needed the national government to build and maintain roads, to enforce contracts, and to organize an educational system. Through the years, this list of requirements for governmental action has been vastly expanded, but that expansion has consistently been justified in Adam Smith's terms—as provisions necessary to ensure the just and free working of the market. Analagously, when individuals attempt to extend their own lives, they require a substructure—a whole network of decisions about the funding of health-related research, the distribution of health information, the creation and maintenance of health institutions, and the distribution of resources for the purchase of health services.

The right to a prolonged life, however, does not posit a civic obligation to provide all the resources possible for the widespread extension of life. Every individual, for example, does not have a right to be given an artificial heart, nor does every individual have an unlimited claim on hemodialysis facilities. All that is required is that reasonable opportunities for health maintenance be provided from public and private sources, and that these opportunities be fairly distributed.

The justice or fairness of the system of opportunities related to health maintenance should be considered on at least two levels: (1) with reference to the allocation of resources for research and services in health-related fields; and (2) with reference to the distribution of resources among various groups within the population. On the first level, justice requires that a wide spectrum of social claims receives fair attention in the distribution of public funds and energies. We need to consider, therefore, whether the area of health is being treated fairly in relation to the other areas. As a start, some random figures may help us to visualize the amount of resources currently being devoted to longevity-supporting medical activities. For example, approximately 9 percent of the gross national product is directed to health costs—a figure that includes an allocation of about one-eighth of the total federal budget. In the years after World War II, $1 of ever $22 were spent by Americans for health services; today $1 of $12 will go for that purpose. Each year $1 billion is being spent on hemodialysis and kidney transplants alone; $250 million, on suturing material; and $112 million, on hypodermic needles (Cohn and Milius 1980).

I am not suggesting that mistakes are being made. I am suggesting, though, that extremely large amounts of money are already being devoted toward activities supportive of longevity, and that justice requires this allocation to be evaluated constantly in light of competitive social needs. There are limits. Our society may never fully be involved in a sum-zero game, where funds going to health care and research literally reduce allocations to education, the development of alternative sources of energy, water resources, or welfare support for the blind and the otherwise disabled. But in a national economy where, for various structural reasons, growth is not what it used to be, we may find ourselves thinking more and more in sum-zero terms. How important, after all, are health services as compared to educational services? How much money ought to be devoted to energy? To the military? How many hours and dollars should be given to children as compared with hours and dollars for elderly people? How do we decide? What are the mechanisms within which people cast their votes?

The second level for inquiry relates to the distribution of resources among various classes of citizens. We should seriously consider, for example, whether the folk saying that claims that "rich people age well" is accurate. Those who believe that rich people enter old age with advantages argue that a problem of justice is thereby raised. Wealth gives access to a variety of social and service opportunities; wealth allows for the purchase of interesting experiences; wealth enables the luxury of regular and skilled medical services; wealth makes possible the consumption of balanced, wholesome foods; wealth allows for the accumulation of longevity-enhancing information; and wealth encourages a hunger for education, which in turn opens up a wide range of interests in the later years of life. Assuming for a moment that, on the whole, rich people really do age better than poor people, is the situation fair?

From one perspective, it surely is. As Robert Nozick argues forcefully in his *Anarchy, State, and Utopia* (1968), people are entitled to the benefits of what they have accumulated, as long as they have not accumulated things fraudulantly or by injuring others. But from another perspective, the answer must be that it is not fair. For example, John Rawls (1971), Nozick's colleague at Harvard, counters Nozick's argument by pointing out that people should not necessarily be rewarded because they were born with native intelligence or because they inherited their father's business, or because their families were blessed with wealthy parents or grandparents.

To follow Rawls's general argument is to conclude that the public right to prolonged life necessarily involves a bias toward the poor or people who are handicapped in various other ways. Rawls adamantly insists that he is not in favor of leveling social classes. But he does believe that particular attention should be given to the people who are worst off. They deserve compensatory services in order to place them in a better position to compete more effectively for the primary goods of life, including life itself.

Indeed, John Rawls's argument seems to take us straight to an assertion that the right to a prolonged life involves the guarantee of some minimum level of medical care for all American citizens. What that minimum should be, of course, is open to debate. Would it include the right to organ transplants? Would it involve, in the case of the elderly, a right to publicly supported care in well-equipped nursing facilities? Would it guarantee an artificial limb? The obvious point is that any specified floor of medical care would have to include some things and not others. The decision as to which things would be provided would have to be based on some intuitive estimate concerning what is fair, in light of all the competitive demands on public funds.

When Rawls's argument is used to interpret the right to a prolonged life, in fact, the justice of some potentially guaranteed level of income (in addition to a guaranteed floor of medical services) is also raised for consideration. If "the rich age well" in any sense, perhaps the poor require a state-secured base of the longevity-supporting goods that money buys. Not all of these goods are medical. Man does not live by medical services alone, but also by education, economic self-respect, mobility, and engagement in community affairs. The issue of whether to establish a guaranteed annual income is, of course, just as explosive in America as the issue of whether to guarantee some level of health service for everyone. Both proposals suggest major redistributions of income. Both are represented in some quarters as the very embodiment of justice and in others as potentially satanic violations of legitimate government functions—the confiscation of money that has been earned honestly in order to transfer it to nondeserving people.

We need to have a lively political discussion about Rawls's provocative proposals, if only to clarify our thinking about what justice requires. Certainly we have little agreement in America about what forms of support are required by the right to a prolonged life. We have committed ourselves to generous support of the research war against disease, and, with some notable exceptions, to the provision of expensive drugs, machines, and services for all persons who are in imminent danger of death. The medical profession, the research establishment, and the general public have, by and large, come to agree that society has a responsibility to fight the agents of death. The resultant war against death involves transfers of money as the tax system takes from some and gives to others. But so far the transfers have not been experienced as damaging because the body politic is content with the obligation that disease and death must be conquered.

What the body politic is not yet content with is Rawls's idea that the right to a prolonged life may involve a systematic, institutionalized responsibility for the minimum conditions of sustained health and welfare. This is an issue, or rather a set of issues, that must inevitably surface as the American public faces the prospect of an increasingly aged population in the context of a less-than-bouyant economy. That it will surface is virtually assured by the militancy of groups like the Gray Panthers, who know that problems of fairness will be argued mainly when they can no longer be kept out of sight. In the political arena, might does not make right; but the political organization of persons who feel themselves to be oppressed does serve to keep alive the civic debate about what justice requires. It is undoubtedly in the ferment created by the militancy of the elderly that the fuller meaning of the right to a prolonged life will be explored.

IS THERE A RIGHT TO A "FULL" LIFE?

In the story of Eos and Tithonus, the lesson Eos had to learn was that sheer bodily survival is not a worthy goal. The quest for an immortality devoid of the conditions that give life value is a quest that ultimately becomes obscene. What Eos really wanted was an eternally youthful Tithonus—a Tithonus forever aflame with passion. Romance was the experience that brought meaning to Eos's life, and to have an immortal Tithonus incapable of romance was to gain no victory at all. Indeed, in an alternate version of the myth, Eos transforms her lover into a grasshopper rather than endure him as a babbling reminder of the meaninglessness of physical survival.

Long life is not necessarily the same thing as a full life. The desire to live a long life is a worthy motivation, but what people want is far more than survival—a simple extension of minutes, hours, days, weeks, and months. Perhaps it is true that when confronted with death, people characteristically resist giving up life, no matter how impoverished. But the desire for long life is normally identical with the desire for a full life, a life that is experienced as significant and as productive of a wide range of satisfactions.

For Eos and Tithonus, the full life was conceived as a life of romance, which required, in their eyes, both infinite time and infinite youthfulness. For others, the full life takes such other forms as civic service, family, creativity, work, reflection, worship, friendship, or even, in extreme cases, solitude. As the psychologist Alfred Adler has pointed out, people live with sharply differing images of who they are, what the world is like, what is good and beautiful, and what it takes to live a rich and satisfying life. We live—almost—in different worlds. Certainly everyone has had the experience of being shocked to discover that what seems obviously to be absurd or ugly is valued dearly by someone else. We have all, for example, marveled privately at a friend's choice of an ugly and unenjoyable mate, only to realize that the friend is enjoying the love affair of the century. Many of us also have lectured our children about their grievous errors of judgment, only later to recognize that we have really been trying to impose arbitrarily our own private sets of values. The full life takes many forms, and part of the wisdom of growing old is in learning to be tolerant of the choices other people make.

It is, by the way, this diversity that so baffles gerontologists in their attempts to recognize and measure "successful aging." Although very few philosophers over the centuries have come to the conclusion that the good life is necessarily one that produces self-satisfaction, gerontologists have largely contented themselves with saying that those who have aged successfully are the ones who report contentment with their own lives. Thus, from the point of view of Western thought about ethics, gerontologists have characteristically come close to adopting a softly hedonistic and egoistic definition of the full life—a doctrine that suggests that the full (or successful) life is measured by the ability of that life to provide pleasure for the individual. At best, this is an arbitrary definition; some would say that it is superficial. But what is a gerontologist to do?

Granted that people choose different images of the full life, it cannot be reasonably argued that people have a *right* to such a life. The right to a prolonged life, which can be supported to some degree by public policy, does not necessarily involve the right to a full life. To have a right is legitimately to place a legal or a moral claim on the behavior of others. Rights imply obligations, and obligations are secured only when they are institutionalized.

The full life "happens" for individuals through a combination of factors only partly of their own making. People often choose, for example, to measure the success of their lives in terms of happy marriages, but mates die. People who think of themselves primarily as workers can be victimized by the loss of jobs or by the outmoding of their skills. And people who picture themselves as lovers find themselves threatened by the loss of their fellow romancers. Eos had no established right to a full life. For her the full life required a youthful Tithonous, and after her fatal blunder, she lost her power to secure the conditions that her own version of the satisfying life required.

Nevertheless, it is possible to identify certain conditions that commonsensically belong to the full life, and it seems rational to argue that elderly people informally, if not legally, have a claim to these conditions. For example, people have a need for participation in a web of human relationships—to be included in a community. A kind of violation of rights sometimes occurs when elderly people become isolated, especially when they are cut off from significant human contacts in sometimes less-than-humane nursing homes, or when, after being expelled from the worlds of work and family, they feel they no longer have a place in the significant institutions of human society. Likewise, people need to be acknowledged as valuable, and a kind of violation of rights occurs when elderly people are stigmatized by virtue of their age. The protection from dehumanizing situations cannot be totaly legislated. It can be made the subject of consciousness raising, however, and it can be identified among the goals sought by militant movements devoted to the interests of the elderly.

My greatest fear, however, is that the growing size of the elderly population in this nation may actually reduce the likelihood that they can experience the full life, or even a humane life, simply because the needs of this elderly population may seem to conflict with the needs of other groups. We may soon be in a situation, for example, where the elimination of mandatory retirement will be viewed as directly precluding younger people from the labor market. Burdens placed on the Social Security system may be seen as a tangible threat to an equally secure future for the young. And the pension systems for public workers may be viewed as the occasion for civic bankruptcy. In these circumstances, the conditions for a new and virulent prejudice against the elderly seem unmistakably to be present.

We are entering a period when people who believe that the right to a prolonged life implies a *claim* to the full life need to be wary. They need to recognize that the situation is inflammatory, and that advocacy of elderly rights may conflict with veiled but severe forms of opposition. Leadership in this period will require a heightened sensitivity not only to the peculiar needs of elderly people, whose claims to a full life may increasingly be undermined, but also to the rights of other groups.

The rights of the elderly are terribly important, but they do not constitute the single priority in American life. The interests of the elderly in preserving the conditions of a full life will be best protected in a just society, where the interests of all groups have been effectively represented and at least tolerably reconciled.

THE NEED FOR A GOOD DEATH

The psychologist Robert Jay Lifton has argued (1971) that the American public, caught in an era of dizzying social change, yearns for immortality and seeks it in the transcendent experience of nature, in meditational disciplines, and in dogmatic attachments to political, religious, and social movements. To this list we should probably add our perennial quest for an actual bodily longevity through research, medical care, and health maintenance programs.

Americans seem to be a people impoverished by an inability to handle the fact of death, and thus lacking an intuitive sense of life's boundedness. For Lifton, this sense of boundedness, of finitude, is associated with the experience of personal significance—the affirmation that one's commitments, one's involvements in the human community constitute urgent matters for decision, because they all must be established in the confines of a finite life span. Assuming that Lifton's arguments are valid, as I believe they are, the right to a prolonged, full life needs the qualifying idea of imminent death.

Life lived without a feeling for the boundaries of birth and death, without the hope of a culminating contribution, or without the possibility of a climactic moment in the life story, is a superficial and incomplete life. Perhaps the primary contribution of the gods to Eos was the gift of helping her to recognize that death plays an important role for human beings in creating the very possibility of a well-crafted life.

This is also the contribution of the rather strange and intense preoccupation with death and dying that has been so visible in the American press and in the university classroom during the recent past. Such a fascination may in fact indicate the public need to balance the culturally frenetic search for immortality. The denial of death that Robert Jay Lifton describes as a modern American tendency cannot be sustained. People need to die. Just as important, people need to know they will die. A good death, an anticipated death, a death visualized as being in good season, a death that may even contribute to the welfare of others—if not a right, this is certainly an element of a richly fulfilled life.

We can only hope that Eos learned her lessons well. It was just as important for Tithonus to die as it was for him to live. And it was more beautiful to have the memories of romance than it was frustratedly to wish that the days of youth might continue forever. Eos had done a good thing. She had used all her powers to gain a long and full life for the person she loved. She ultimately failed, but she also won, because she was able to add to her understanding of the human condition. Her heightened insight is her gift to us, and we should be grateful to her.

REFERENCES

Cohn, Victor, and Peter Milius. 1980. "Medicine 1980: The View from the *Washington Post*." *Forum* 3:27.

Evelyn-White, Hugh G., trans. 1914. *Hesiod, Homeric Hymns and Homerica*. New York: Loeb Classical Library.

Frazer, James G. 1918. *Folk-Lore in the Old Testament*, vol. I. London: MacMillan.

Lifton, Robert Jay. 1971. *History and Human Survival*. New York: Random House. (See especially his essay on "Protean Man," pp. 311–331.)

Nozick, Robert. 1968. *Anarchy, State, and Utopia*. New York: Basic Books. (See especially Chapter 7.)

Percival, Thomas. "Of Professional Conduct." In *Ethics in Medicine*, edited by Stanley Joel Reiser, Arthur Dyk, and William Curran, p. 19. Cambridge, Mass.: MIT Press.

Rawls, John. 1971. *A Theory of Justice*. Cambridge, Mass.: Harvard University Press. (See especially Chapter 2.)

"Selections from the Hippocratic Corpus." In *Ethics in Medicine*, edited by Stanley Joel Reiser, Arthur Dyk, and William Curran, p. 6. Cambridge, Mass.: MIT Press.

Smith, Adam, 1937. *The Wealth of Nations*. New York: Random House.

IV UNIVERSITY OF WASHINGTON WORLD PERSPECTIVES ON AGING

INTRODUCTION
Alice J. Kethley

The 1970s have been described by many as the decade in which "aging" came of age: at least within the United States, aging and the aged became focal points in a number of major arenas during that time. Congress, state legislatures, and local governments devoted time and money attempting to pass sound legislation for service programs, Medicare and Medicaid, and Social Security. Clichés such as the "graying of the federal budget" became common. Throughout the nation colleges and universities initiated academic programs to train gerontologists and geriatric clinicians, to conduct research, and to study the aging process. Popular literature, current-event magazines, academic journals, and newspapers reflected a dramatic increase in writings on aging. A relatively new and very large job market developed for professionals and paraprofessionals in nursing homes, social service agencies, retirement communities, senior centers, and a wide variety of health care agencies. Perhaps the most powerful indication came from the elderly themselves, who for the first time in large numbers joined national or state organizations with age as the major criterion for membership. Some of these organizations not only provided special benefits to their members, but also developed into recognized political influ-

231

ences. Senior lobby groups and silver-haired legislatures became common in almost every state.

This national consciousness raising has brought benefits but also liabilities, as the process has tended to emphasize the problems of the elderly. On the positive side, retired individuals have changed our perceptions about older people's ability to organize on their own behalf and act in their own interest. In a society that has been characterized as youth oriented, gray became beautiful and a more positive trend in attitude began to emerge. On the negative side, the extreme tactics necessary to convince government and the public of the need for better benefits and expanded programs for the elderly have led many to view them as a social and economic liability. The tendency has been to blame the elderly rather than to recognize that programs such as Social Security and Medicare are in need of revision.

The consciousness raising of the seventies has culminated with the recognition that extension of life has increased the numbers of older individuals, and this in turn has led to a multiplicity of new issues. These issues cannot be legislated away. Neither can they be treated or cured. Dollars and services merely mask the symptoms of underlying problems. Aging must be recognized as a normal process to which most of us aspire, and it carries with it a host of benefits as well as problems. The lesson of the seventies is the need for a partnership between the elderly and the other members of society, if indeed the later years are to be the "greater years."

The 1980s must be a decade of action and solutions. The statistics and numbers that were so much a part of the new awareness raising are no longer impressive. The needs have been assessed and recognized. The more relevant question at this point is: "What will be our course of action?"

"World Perspectives on Aging," a public lecture series presented by the University of Washington's Institute on Aging and supported by Colonial Penn Insurance Group, had as its overall objective to provide the Seattle community—retired persons, students, academics, and professionals—with an opportunity to broaden their understanding of aging. It was an attempt to change our focus on the problems of aging by considering them, not as an artifact of U.S. industrialization and modernization, but rather as a phenomenon with global implications. Using a lecture-and-question format, the series presented information on other nations and showed how they are addressing the issues with which we struggle. The series also attempted to present both the more pragmatic issues—through "Social Policy in Aging"—and equally important but less tangible influences—through "A Philosophy of Aging from a World Perspective" and "Cultural Influences in Aging." A world perspective was chosen in recognition that, although the United States has experienced dramatic population shifts, there are indeed other nations which have experienced the same or even more dramatic shifts, reflected in either percentages or sheer numbers. We anticipated that a great deal could be learned by examining the social, political, and philosophical strategies of other nations.

Because health is a top concern of this nation's elderly, it was chosen as a topic for discussion in this published lecture series. The topic was expanded to include social services in recognition that individuals need both medical and social care. Indeed it seems a bureaucratic and professional convenience that the two have been separated. The nearly universal development of health care and social service systems characterizes the worldwide concern for the well-being of older persons. The range of national strategies varies greatly, reflecting the cultural, economic, and political structures of each nation. Countries with strong family systems, such as Thailand, have structured their services around the family. Nations such as the United States with its highly industrialized economy, nuclear families, and high respect for specialists and experts, have developed systems centered around such trained professionals as medical doctors, nurses, and social workers.

Actions and policies also embody an underlying philosophy. By and large, those of us involved in what we consider to be scientific problem solving tend to ignore the field that has been known classically as philosophy. Only with a great deal of hesitancy was the subject included in this series, which attracts audiences who are heavily involved with more pragmatic issues. It would have been negligent to have ignored it, however. Michel Philibert's "A Philosophy of Aging from a World Perspective" presents a true global and historical perspective that will enrich each person's individual educational experience. His eloquent presentation includes quotes from scientists, playwrights, philosophers, politicians, and others, and he integrates them into a meaningful discussion of our efforts to classify our own aging into a lucid science-gerontology. Philosophical considerations are indeed essential to a world perspective.

Dr. Erdman Palmore began his presentation with a story not included in his chapter, "Cultural Influences on Aging." The story will be repeated here because it so clearly explains why it is necessary to include culture when considering aging from any perspective:

> Here is a story that comes from China. It's not a funny story, but I think it's a profound one. It concerns a grandfather who lived with his son and his grandson in a poor, remote region of China. One year the harvest was so bad that there was not enough food to go around, and they began slowly to starve. And the old man, who was very, very old, got weaker and weaker because there was so little food for them to eat. Finally the son decided that since his grandfather was so very old, and didn't have long to live anyway, it would be better if he sacrificed his life so that his son and grandson might not starve and would be able to get through the winter. So the son built a bamboo basket big enough to put the grandfather in, and they put the grandfather in the basket, and the son and the grandson carried the basket with the grandfather down to the river. There they said goodbye to the grandfather and dumped him in the river. As they turned to go back, the grandson picked up the basket and started to carry it back with them. His father said, "Why are you carrying that basket back, son?" And the son said, "To use on you when you get old, father."

Dr. Palmore's presentation discusses the impact of U.S. culture in shaping attitudes and policies on aging and creates a conceptual framework for understanding cultural influences on gerontology in other countries.

The actions that any nation takes are determined by its political structure, regardless of how simple or sophisticated it is. Government, which historically has been more concerned with war and power than with social welfare, has universally been forced to address the needs of its citizens of all ages. As Walter Beattie points out in his "Social Policies and Aging: A Global

Perspective," the newest and fastest-growing population group in all nations—especially the less developed ones—is the elderly. Professor Beattie's presentation includes an overview of the development of social security programs, charts of demographic trends, and a candid discussion of what policymakers worldwide are doing to address the issues. He points out that the United Nations' decision to hold a World Assembly on the Elderly in 1982 reflects the concern that all nations feel for their growing population of aged individuals.

Over the past decade, the goal of extended life has become a reality, with life expectancy at birth going up in all nations. Contrary to the myths espoused earlier by individuals like Spain's Ponce de León, the accomplishment of longevity has not been a "fountain of youth." Indeed the reality includes a body and mind that fully reflect the accumulation of the events of one's life. For some, that means chronic illnesses, poverty, immobility, dementia, isolation, and final years in an institution. For others, it means adapting to normal age changes, but without disabilities, disease, or poverty. For the societies of the world it means accommodating to a relatively new population group, some of whom will be dependent citizens in need of health care, economic assistance, and other means of support. As the following pages demonstrate, it is not a simple challenge. It is one which calls for joint planning, as nations throughout the world address the issue of what to do with their "living history"—the elderly among them who have built the foundation of the present.

The problems so clearly recognized in the 1970s by the United States are world problems indeed, and it is appropriate that we take an attitude which includes "World Perspectives on Aging."

12 A PHILOSOPHY OF AGING FROM A WORLD PERSPECTIVE

Michel Philibert

All of us share confused, often contradictory, attitudes about aging. What we have heard, seen, and experienced; what we have said and done about aging, our own and others', has been accumulated and revised throughout our lives.

If philosophy is a way of thinking or living, by which people attempt to reexamine what life has done to them and what they are doing with their lives, we might conceive a philosophy of aging as such an attempt, aiming to reappraise and reorganize our attitudes on aging. It is an attempt to clarify, in a Kantian sense, what we can know about aging, what we must do with our own and others' aging, what we may hope for and expect from aging.

The links between aging and philosophy are both ancient and primitive. In the past, humans have either naively believed, or cleverly so patterned their lives, that they would grow wiser as they grew older. However, they sometimes discovered this was not always the case; that living longer did not spontaneously or necessarily bring wisdom along. "If thou wert my fool, nuncle," says the Fool to King Lear, "I'd have thee beaten for being old before thy time.—How's that?—Thou should'st not have been old till thou hadst been wise." Philosophy emerged as a methodical way of thinking and as a dedicat-

237

ed way of life during one of these historical periods when humanity understood it could grow older without becoming any the wiser, and die a fool. To reach wisdom required planning, discipline, and management.

Some people may well consider philosophy as an obsolescent, even obsolete, discipline. They may think the world no longer needs a "philosophy" of aging; that we may have problems with aging, but Western nations have equipped us with modern, adequate tools to deal with these problems. In this century we have developed *gerontology* as a scientific knowledge of aging, *geriatrics* and *national policies for aging* as sophisticated strategies for managing the aged. These are not merely newly coined labels, but vast new social institutions all geared up and funded to help us manage our problems with aging, old age, and the aged. So why bother with a "philosophy"?

My own contention is that we need such a philosophy more than ever before. Recent, unprecedented changes in the human experience of aging have made obsolete our traditional life patterns and our former ways of managing aging. Our thinking about aging is more confused and more negative than it ever was. Gerontology, geriatrics, and policies for aging are the answers put forward by science and society to face the challenges of our present experience of aging. But they are young, tentative, and inevitably misleading answers. Far from solving our problems, they have further complicated them. Far from rendering a philosophy of aging unnecessary, they feed it with more incentives and make the task only more urgent.

A GLOBAL PERSPECTIVE ON AGING

Over the past two centuries, our experience of aging has been transformed primarily by two types of changes. The first is quantitative: an increase in average human longevity, and an increase in the proportion of the aged in the total population. The second is qualitative: a generalized devaluation of old age and a pervasive fear of aging, of one's own aging. We have already seen such changes transform the experience of aging in the Western, developed nations, and it is probable that similar changes will affect human aging over the next two decades in the developing countries.

During the past two centuries, the average longevity in the West has practically doubled, rising from about thirty-five to seventy years. This has resulted from a sharp decrease in infantile and juvenile mortality rates. For the first time in recorded history, the greater part of all children born alive are (at least in the West) surviving into old age. In eighteenth century France, for example, out of 10,000 children born alive, 5,800 survived at the age of five, and 119 to the age of eighty-five. As of today, out of 10,000 girls born alive, 5,234 will be still living at age eighty, and over 3,000 will still be living beyond eighty-five (Girard 1979). Old age, which throughout history was a rare blessing or an exceptional achievement, has all of a sudden been made accessible to the many.

In about the same period of time, the percentage of people sixty years and over in the living population of the West has been multiplied by four or five times, while the percentage of people under twenty has dropped from over 50 percent of the population to about 30 percent. In France, Great Britain, and Germany, one person out of five is now sixty or over. The overall result of these two combined quantitative changes has been a rapid and unprecedented increase, in the West, of both the numbers and the percentages of older persons now living.

Along with these quantitative changes have come qualitative changes, no less important and unprecedented; and they too have been affecting the experience of human aging. These qualitative changes are more difficult to appraise and to document than the quantitative; they vary more widely according to geographic milieu, social class, cultural tradition, and ethnic group. Overall, however, over the past century the Western nations have experienced a strong devaluation of old age. Once respected or envied as a blessing or a dignity, old age now appears as a burden both to the individual and to the community. We have made age an object of fear, contempt, rejection, an object of pity and condescending care.

Still worse, a rampant fear of aging has developed in the West. Some call it *gerontophobia*, some *ageism*. I prefer to call it *gerascophobia* (from the Greek "gerasco," meaning "I age") in order to stress that it is not only a fear of aging in general, but a fear of one's own aging. This fear has not only contaminated our minds, but also has inhibited or distorted the very growth of our souls. Erik Erikson wrote in 1963: "Healthy children will not fear life if their elders have integrity enough not to fear death," and Montaigne before him (1595) observed that "not to dislike dying is properly becoming only to those who like living." But we have developed such fears of aging and dying that many of our children are reluctant to grow up and grow older. To borrow the terms of Grace Louks Elliot (1964), when "both individuals and society are cheated of the privileges and gifts of old age and death," how shall we "help both the young and the old accept age and death as the fulfillment of life?"

The end result of these quantitative and qualitative changes is that we have simultaneously managed to add years to the human life, and to deprive most of these added years of life, zest, and meaning. As Barbara Anderson (1979) puts it: "Only man among the species applies such consummate skill to the social destruction of his own membership at the same time as he pursues, with scientific relentlessness, the prolongation of life itself. It makes no sense."

All demographic forecasts make it a near certainty that in the next two or three decades the developing countries, which are already affected by a decrease in both infantile mortality rates and fecundity, will experience a resulting increase both in the percentage and in the number of their older population. This quantitative change will be similar to that which happened in the West, only more rapid and shattering. The report of the Secretary General of the United Nations on *Problems of the Elderly and the Aged* (March 13, 1980) points out that in 1970 there were 307 million persons over sixty years of age in the world, and that by the year 2000 this number will grow to nearly 580 million—an increase of nearly 90 percent. In the developing regions, the older population will increase by approximately 123 percent.

Will the qualitative changes in Western attitudes toward aging—the devaluation of old age, the devastating fear of aging—inevitably accompany these quantitative changes in the rest of the world? Will they be fatal? Can we but wait and see?

Or can we now design a strategy that will save humankind from choking to death on its own fear of aging and dying? If humankind has a chance to find new ways of getting wiser and living longer, must it be now or never?

Before developing tentative answers to these questions, two possible misunderstandings must be prevented. The first would be to think that we should aim our efforts at preserving in the developing countries the traditional life-course patterns, social rituals, and cultural concepts that stress the positive aspects of human aging and provide compensations for its inevitable losses and decrements. However, this would be a mistake. Such traditional patterns are already disrupted and might entirely collapse in one or two generations as industrialization, urbanization, science, and technology tighten their networks over the world. Traditional ways of thinking will resist only for a time the breakdown of traditional modes and conditions of living. We can neither preserve nor restore rituals and philosophies of the past, however adequate they were for centuries.

A second and much more dangerous misunderstanding would be to think that gerontology, geriatrics, and policies on aging are already providing us with sound answers to the problems of human aging. Over the past thirty years we have developed in Europe and North America a network of gerontological societies, institutes, centers, programs, meetings, curricula, diplomas, honors, awards, grants, journals, libraries, laboratories; of geriatrics centers, homes, personnel, training, drugs, props; of administrations on aging, Golden Age clubs, senior citizen centers, retirement homes and villages, old-age pensions, social policies, Third Age universities, a gray lobby, an aging enterprise, and so on and on. They provide us with travel expenses, jobs, careers, fame, power, prestige, and the ego-comforting delusion that we are useful. We may be tempted to think that only by further developing our gerontological programs, and by teaching the developing countries to copy our strategies, will we overcome the challenge of aging. I am of the opposite persuasion. It would be detrimental, perhaps even fatal, for the rest of the world to uncritically duplicate the current Western misconceptions and mismanagement of human aging.

AN EVALUATION OF CURRENT
GERONTOLOGY AND POLICIES ON AGING

The most fundamental misconception in current gerontology has to do with its view of aging as a natural, biological deterioration of the living organism over time, leading to its death. This view leads to a conception (or misconception) of gerontology as a scientific investigation of aging, which measures and explains impairment and losses of functions, diminishing capacities for adjustment, and assesses their phases, causes, mechanisms, and laws.

When I call these views "misconceptions," I am not denying the existence of natural and specific processes of changes over time in the different living species. Neither am I denying the detrimental character of several of these changes, nor the legitimacy of their scientific investigation. What I am denying is the idea that in any living species, and especially humans, the detrimental aspects of some of these changes support a concept of aging as one essentially destructive process. Such a view is biologically unsound and misleading; furthermore, to reduce human aging to its natural aspects is anthropologically unsound, a fallacy.

Biologically, aging means growing older, living longer. There is no escape from death, but aging. There is no escape from aging, but dying at once. Our only alternative to an early death is to age. Far from being a process leading to my death, aging is the process of living longer, of postponing further the execution of the death sentence impending since the day I was conceived. We must apply to aging the definition that Xavier Bichat (1800) gave of life, and see it as "the ensemble of functions that resist death." Biologically, aging must be investigated as a longer sustained victory of life over death.

More fundamental than the biological misconception of aging as a destructive process is the anthropological misconception that reduces human aging to a natural process. Man is indeed an animal. But the science of man that began with Aristotle must focus again today on identifying the specific traits, if any, which distinguish our species from other living species. When we look at man as a rational animal, a political animal, a speaking animal, a laughing animal, a storytelling animal, a self-interpreting animal, we are on the right track. When Leo Simmons said that man is the only animal that can be persuaded to take care of his grandfather; when Linden and Courtney (1953) argue that the older person has responsibilities not found among other animals because human societies require an extended period of socialization of the young, and a complex means of preserving and communicating the heritage of society; when Barbara Anderson (1979) angrily observes that only man among the species applies such consummate skill to the social destruction of his own membership—such statements make gerontology a specifically human science.

Whenever current gerontology fails to take into account the specificity of human animals, it regresses from science to scientific ideology or to plain ideology. Yet what puzzles the philosopher most is how seldom and how few gerontologists address the issue of the specificity of human aging. Although many authors of gerontological works include the word "human" in their title, none bothers to raise the question of its specificity. However, if we want to make gerontology a science, not an ideology—if we want to develop a *human gerontology*— we should ground our studies on the specificity of human aging. Man dies as other animals do. But man is aware of having to die: other animals are not. Man ages as other animals do. But man is aware of aging, and to that extent he does not age quite like other animals do. He either fears aging or looks forward to it. Man observes aging, discusses it, speculates and fantasizes about it. He assumes or denies it. He makes the best or the worst of it.

Such uniquely human responses make it all the more necessary to revise our very definition of aging. In all living species, changes over time may happen either as programmed by nature, according to a pattern that is the same for all the members of each species, or as a result of varying circumstances that differently affect individuals or subcategories. At first it seems reasonable to use the term "aging" to label only the series of changes that appear to be universal in a given species, and therefore natural. And indeed most gerontologists have done exactly this, implicitly or explicitly assuming that one must investigate human aging as a natural process. But the changes that affect man over time do not all result from either

Figure 12–1   Ambivalence of Aging

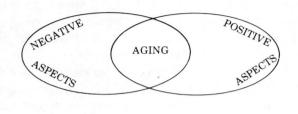

AMBIVALENCE OF AGING

FORCES ACTIVE IN AND ON AGING

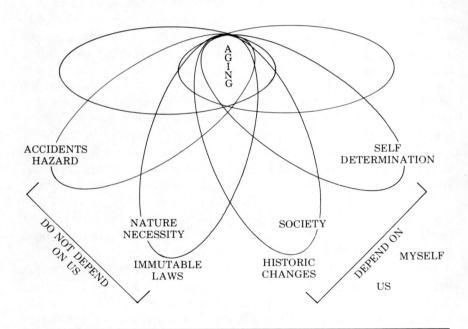

natural causes or accidents. Some result from the way a society is organized and functions; some others result from our own
action—they are self-induced changes.

At a first glance it seems that puberty or menopause are
age-related changes, whereas learning Latin or painting, or going abroad, may be undertaken at any age and therefore must

not be included in an investigation of aging as such. Here is precisely the point at which I take my leave from current gerontology. Learning and traveling are activities that indeed we may indulge in at different ages; but their pattern and efficiency may vary widely according to the age at which we get started, and also at the moment in history when we are practicing them. Moreover our progress or decline, our achievements and failures in such activities will stretch over a longer or shorter time; they will follow some sort of sequential pattern; they will consolidate, accumulate, maintain themselves, or deteriorate over time.

The changes that affect my life over time may originate in nature, in fortune, in society, or in my own activity: but all are to develop and to combine their consequences as time goes on, as the waters from different sources unite and mix to form one and the same river. For all species, aging means growing older and living longer; but aging for humans also means learning— and unlearning—longer, changing longer, and integrating through time all the changes that we either undergo or initiate (see Figure 12–1). And the experience of human aging is not only given to us by nature: it is also interpreted and managed by us.

Therefore, an investigation of the natural changes that affect us over time, while important, cannot explain our experience of aging: they provide only one set of components among others, and are interpreted in the broader context of our experience. And our experience of aging, interpreted and managed by us, calls for an investigation of its own, which can restrict itself neither to the objects nor to the methods of the natural sciences.

Social institutions and cultural rules, on the one hand, and individual decisions, on the other, interfere over time with the changes that either nature or fortune brings about in our lives. A resulting specific trait of human aging, as compared with aging in other species, is the endless variation of its patterns and styles. They vary from one individual to another, from one group to another, from one historical period to another. Age changes and historic changes are woven into one and the same design. The variations in human aging make it much more

plastic and versatile than in any other species. Another specific trait of human aging results from its ambivalence: it may be
easy or difficult, good or bad. Open to interpretation, amenable
to management, flexible to social and to personal interven-
tions, human aging may be patterned for the better or for the
worse.

Paul Ricoeur once wrote: "Life for humans is a complex,
knotty situation, an unsolved problem. Thus it is an open question confronting the will. It is why finally there is a problem of
choice and a moral problem." Aging for humans is also a complex, knotty course of change, an unsolved problem—and
therefore an open question confronting the will. That is why
gerontology cannot restrict its task to observing facts but has
to interpret and intervene. That is why policies on aging must
go beyond social programs and administrative strategies, beyond conflicting economic interests and political forces: aging
implies a moral choice and ethical principles. That is why both
gerontology and policies on aging can grow to their full size
only in the broader frame of a philosophy of aging, which links
together the epistemological question raised by gerontology:
What can we know about aging?—the ethical question raised
by our policies on aging: What must we do about aging?—and
the third question, existential or metaphysical: What may we
hope for, and expect from, aging?

One further sign of the specificity of human aging comes
from Charles Taylor's definition (1971) of man as a self-interpreting animal. The experience of human aging is not only an
object for interpretation: it is also a *process* of interpretation.
An unexamined, an unexamining, aging is not worth living.
Aging offers to all humans the possibility—and to those who
grasp it, the capacity—of continually renewing their interpretation and redirection of life.

Think, for example, of any past action or event that has
been important in your life, be it your first pair of pants or
your first holy communion, the death of a dear one or your
first kiss, or when you left home for college, had an abortion or
an accident, won the race, were given an award, or were
mugged in the street. It does not matter whether you think of
a short event, like your first kiss, a longer one like your honey-
moon, or even your marriage if you are now divorced. The only

requirement is that you think of a past event or sequence, something that now is over. In doing so you have already interpreted that action or event at least three times: before it happened, while it was happening, and after it had happened.

Before it happened, you were anticipating it, planning on it, preparing for it. You were interpreting the event, giving it a pattern and a meaning, finally making up your mind. And then it happened: you lived through it. It was certainly more or less different from what you had been expecting, and you kept comparing the way it was with the way you had thought it would be. You were surprised; you were disappointed, or fulfilled beyond expectation. So you had to adapt to the happening, to revise your schemes, to work out a different interpretation. You found a new meaning—a second one.

And then it was over. You left your parents, buried your father, sold the house, gave up racing, lost your job, received your pardon, parted from your spouse. Whenever you look at this past period of your life in retrospect, it appears once more as different from both your first anticipation and from the actual experience. Consequences have since developed that you had not foreseen at the time, and they have changed the very meaning of the past event. You now use different criteria to appraise your past deeds, to weigh your gains and your losses. Some of your past successes, so exhilarating when you first achieved them, now appear as the beginning of your decline and fall. Some of your past failures, so hard to take when they happened, you may now count among your blessings. You have with time given a third meaning to the event, which you now see in the new context of what you have been through since that time.

After this third, retrospective interpretation has been worked out and crystallized into a narrative, one of two things may happen as you keep living on. First, having fixed the meaning of the event through your effort at interpretation, you may play it back as many times as occasion will require, as you play a record again and again. You have encapsulated the past in an image so satisfying that you will afterward always refer to that image and repeat your tale, unchanged, till you die. A substitute to your past, the image will become a barrier between you and your life. If this happens, you are not aging well: you are alienated from your own image. But if, on the contrary, you really keep living on—keep learning new things, developing new skills, making new commitments, new friends, new discoveries—you will increase day after day the distance from which you may recall your past experiences, and these past periods of your life will keep changing their meaning and, so to speak, their future. For as long as you keep on living, your past has a future.

You cannot change your past. What is done is done; what is lost is lost; but you may indeed change the meaning of your past. Today and tomorrow you may confirm, betray, or redeem what you have done and been, in the past. Aging therefore provides humans with an opportunity for endlessly reinterpreting their experience of aging; and this work of reinterpretation constitutes this experience and gives meaning to it.

This conception of human aging as endless reinterpretation of experience in the present lays the ground for human gerontology. Since human aging is both an object and a process of interpretation, the method of human gerontology must be interpretive and interventive. As an interpretive process it must borrow its materials, tools, and hypotheses from history, from social anthropology, from cultural geography, from art and literary criticism, from semiotics and hermeneutics. As an interventive process it must look on education, rehabilitation, geriatric medicine, social policies, work and leisure patterns, living conditions, and policies on aging, not only as domains of "applied" gerontology, but as domains in which to test and rejuvenate our current understanding, our current management of human aging.

At present, however, gerontology remains a discipline that has yet to realize the full potential of its subject by viewing aging as an opportunity and the aged as a resource. Gerontology has instead mistaken aging for a natural phenomenon, and has mimicked natural sciences, unwillingly justifying current misconceptions about and mismanagement of, old age.

In part, current gerontological approaches are hampered by excessive reliance on the concept of scientific ideology. As Georges Canguilhem has recently pointed out (1977), in trying to understand the origins of current scientific concepts, the historian looks back to concepts and approaches which preceded those now established and were finally discredited and expelled from the realm of science. Some of these outdated materials—mythical, religious, magical—were never meant as science. Some others were mistaken as scientific. They were borrowed from a preexistent scientific discipline and applied to problems in another realm of experience with the expectation that being scientific in origin and intent, they would provide their new object with an adequate explanation.

But these ready-made thoughts seldom fit the new area to which they are transferred. They need to be amended at the least, and may finally be scrapped altogether as inadequate and misleading. They are no longer part of science; however, something of their insight may still haunt contemporary thinking, which has been worked out with different materials and skills but sometimes along a similar pattern. Canguilhem calls these "scientific ideologies," and to my mind, there have been many of these among the gerontological output over the past decades.

Gerontology has also suffered from the modern conviction that knowledge has become a key to power—power over nature and over our fellow creatures. Scientific activity has therefore become a wage-earning activity and a social institution, to the point where we now have several times more scientists alive, working, and paid for than ever before. Social scientists as well as natural scientists have benefited from the new opportunities for money and fame opened by modern science. Psychologists, sociologists, and gerontologists have been crowding to the expected harvesting.

But it is obvious that the revolution which transformed the natural sciences did not catch the social sciences at the same phase of their theoretical evolution. A high level of intellectual coherency, social agreement, and mutual recognition among scientists had been achieved in the natural sciences before science emerged as a power-producing and fund-raising activity. However, psychology and sociology—and particularly gerontology—have not yet reached the same level. In order to justify the money they use and to court the fame which has crowned the Galileos and Darwins, social scientists have yielded in all good faith to the temptation of designing their methods for the study of man according to models of the sciences of nature that have proved so rewarding in money, prestige, and influence. Instead of patterning their research to focus on the specificity of the human animal, they mimicked the natural sciences and produced scientific ideology in tons of printed paper and hurricanes of words.

Governmental policies on aging have suffered from misperceptions similar to those afflicting the field of gerontology in general. The situation in France provides a typical case in point. French policy over the past two decades has had three main objectives: (1) to provide an income to those who are retired from paid work; (2) to provide health care for the sick, and retirement or nursing homes for the isolated or invalid; (3) to help some 8 percent of those over age sixty-five to stay in their homes when they could no longer do so without help; and to encourage social participation by all retirees in community life. A great deal of money goes to income maintenance; in fact, such funds have doubled in fifteen years and comprise more than twenty times the cost of health care for the aged, and about forty times the cost of social programs for the aged. Income maintenance funds are, however, very unequally distributed; and health care, home care, and homes for the aged are reluctantly funded and inadequately provided. In addition, practically nothing is being done either to adapt working conditions to changes in the individual over time, or to enforce the right of the aged—or even the middle-aged—to work.

These shortcomings reveal the fourth, hidden function of the French policy on aging. In the past two decades, the French government has implicitly assigned to old-age policies the function of slightly adapting, aptly disguising, and secretly consecrating a life course that has arisen spontaneously from unplanned cultural, social, and economic evolution. Historically, an average life course follows three distinct stages. The first is childhood and youth, largely passed in education; the second, which increasingly begins later and ends earlier, dedicated to work; and the third, also increasing at both ends, beginning with an earlier age of retirement and ending later with the increase in life expectancy. In the third stage, social inequalities in education, work, health care, and money accumulate to make old age easier for the socially privileged, but make it a period of deprivation and lowered expectations for most.

In *A Good Age* (1977), Alex Comfort points out that

the things which make oldness insupportable in human societies don't at all commonly arise from consequences of the biological process. They arise from sociogenic aging, i.e. from the role which society imposes on people as they reach a certain chronological age. At this age they retire, or, in plain words, are rendered unemployed, useless, and in some cases, impoverished. After that transition, and in proportion to their chronological age, they are prescribed to be unintelligent, unemployable, crazy and asexual.

Within this context, the French policy on aging has one primary, though hidden, function: it masks the failure or absence of a policy for aging over the life course, one that might aim to redistribute education, work, rewards, rest, recreation, and service over the life span and across social boundaries; to give hope and a future to more people of every age; and to make each step on the human age ladder a higher one.

In contrast to this, gerontology currently suggests that satisfaction in old age should result mainly from adapting oneself to the natural, irreversible, detrimental laws of the aging process, and to the current social organization of our society. No wonder it has reinforced rather than cured our rampant gerascophoby.

The life experience of those humans who now reach old age has been similar to none in the past, and probably to none in the future; in their lifetime mankind and the world have changed more dramatically than ever before. Mankind has gone from its preindustrial stage to the dawn of its postindustrial, ecological age. We have moved from country to city, from the horse to the jet and the missile, from walking to flying, from the semaphore and drum to radio and television. We have acquired more power over the environment and over people than ever before. The aged of today have been both witnesses and partners to these developments. They have been their authors and pioneers, and their victims and beneficiaries.

During this century mankind has acquired and refined two possibilities for committing suicide. The quicker way would be through nuclear war. A slightly longer way in which we are already engaged, is by destroying cultivable soils, wasting nonrenewable resources, polluting the air and oceans, extinguishing thousands of living species, disrupting the ecological balance of life on the planet, and ceasing to give life, to give birth. We perish from clinging to our own life, power, and pride. Earlier on, I quoted Erik Erikson saying, "healthy children will not fear life if their elders have integrity enough not to fear death." We in the West have reached such a point in our fear of aging and dying that we are afraid to give life, to bear children anymore, thus sentencing ourselves to extinction.

In this situation, the aged all over the world might well be our last resource, to help us open our eyes and change our ways before it becomes too late. Thus the work of reinterpreting their experience and redirecting their life is not a private concern as most of us wrongly think; it is a task of utmost importance and meaning. Our problem is not salvaging old age; it is whether we may be salvaged and see our days prolonged by respecting our elders.

Some may object that the more the world has been changing, the more those born a long time ago are outdated and unable to adapt to the changes. I have never thought that a long and rich experience spontaneously coalesces into wisdom. But I do not think either that a lack of experience and easy adaptation to contemporary gadgets necessarily qualifies youth to meet our present challenges. Youth cannot but begin with prejudices; and even if age alone does not overcome our prejudices, we do need time to get rid of some of them. Even though older people are not all wise, they have acquired an experience that we all need, and in neglecting this potential resource we nullify it in them as well as for us.

Where Shakespeare's Fool said we should become wise before becoming old, Marcel Proust, the greater student of aging in this century, takes an even more radical position: that we should reach truth before reaching death. Proust was among the first to articulate aging as concomitant physical decline and spiritual growth, and to link both to suffering, grief, and death. He makes suffering and anticipation of death central to aging, because suffering to him is accountable at the same time for the destructive as well as the creative dimensions of aging:

> Unhappiness ends by killing. . . . But since force of one kind can change into a force of another kind, since heat which is stored up becomes light and the electricity in a flash of lightning can cause a photograph to be taken, since the dull pain in our heart can hoist above itself like a banner the visible permanence of an image for every new grief, let us accept the physical injury which is done to us for the sake of the spiritual knowledge which grief brings. . . . Sufferings are servants, obscure and detested, against whom one struggles, beneath whose dominion one more and more completely falls, dire and dreadful servants whom it is impossible to replace and who by subterranean paths lead us towards truth and death. Happy are those who have first come face to face with truth, those for whom, near though the one may be to the other, the hour of truth has struck before the hour of death! (*Le temps retrouvé.*)

Indeed, Proust's advice might be valid beyond his intention and awareness, not only for the individual, but for us as a species. From a world perspective, at this unique moment in the history of humankind and the spaceship earth, happy will we be if, calling on the aged of today as indispensable partners in our examination of past experience and planning for the future, we may reach truth and wisdom in time to save our species on the planet, instead of falling into our own traps and dying fools.

REFERENCES

Anderson, Barbara Gallatin. 1979. *The Aging Game*. New York: McGraw Hill.

Birren, James E. 1960. *Handbook of Aging and the Individual*. Chicago: University of Chicago Press.

Birren, James E.; R.N. Butler; S.W. Greenhouse; L. Sokoloff; and M.R. Yarrow. 1963. *Human Aging*. Washington, D.C.: Public Health Service (PHS Publication 986).

Birren, James E., and V. Jayne Renner. 1979. "Research on the Psychology of Aging: Principles and Experimentation." In *Handbook of the Psychology of Aging*, edited by J.E. Birren and K. Warner Schaie, pp. 3–28. London: Von Nostrand Reinhold.

Bichat, Xavier. 1800. *Recherches Physiologiques sur la Vie et la Mort.* Paris: Chez Brosson, Gabon et cie.

Binstock, Robert. 1977. "Aging and Public Policy." In *Gerontology at St. Michaels*, edited by Joseph Gaida. Colcester, Vermont: St. Michael's College.

Bromley, Dennis B. 1977. *The Psychology of Human Ageing.* Baltimore: Penguin Books.

Butler, Robert N. 1963. "The Life Review: An Interpretation of Reminiscence in the Aged." In *New Thoughts on Old Age*, edited by Robert Kastenbaum, pp. 265–80. New York: Springer Publishing.

Canguilhem, Georges. 1977. *Ideologie et Rationalité dans l'Histoire des Sciences de la Vie.* Paris: Vrin.

Chown, Sheila, ed. 1972. *Human Ageing.* Baltimore: Penguin Books.

Comfort, Alex. 1956. *The Biology of Senescence*, 1st ed. London: Routledge and Kegan Paul.

Comfort, Alex. 1964. *The Process of Aging.* New York: Signet Science Books.

Comfort, Alex. 1976. *A Good Age.* New York: Crown Publishers.

Comfort, Alex. 1979. *The Biology of Senescence.* 3rd ed. New York: Elsevier North Holland.

Elliot, Grace Louks. *To Come Full Circle. 1964.* Quoted in Doris Webster Havice, "Old Age: The Possibility of Enlightenment." *Soundings* 57:70–79.

Erikson, Erik. 1963. *Childhood and Society*, 2nd ed. New York: W.W. Norton & Co.

Estes, Carroll. 1979. *The Aging Enterprise.* San Francisco: Jossey Bass.

Girard, Alain. 1979. "Le Nouveau Regime Demographique et la Crise des Valeurs." *Les Etudes* 350:7–23.

Guillemard, Anne-Marie. 1980. *La Vieillesse et l'Etat.* Paris: Presses Universitaires Françaises.

Handler, P. 1960. "Radiation and Aging." In *Aging,* edited by Nathan Shock, pp. 199–223. Washington, D.C.: American Association for the Advancement of Science.

Kastenbaum, Robert. 1979. "Loving, Dying, and Other Gerontologic Addendo." In *The Psychology of Adult Development and Aging,* edited by Carl Eisdorfer and M. Powell Lawton, pp. 699–708. Washington, D.C.: American Psychological Association.

Koch, Kenneth. 1977. *I've Never Told Anybody.* New York: Random House.

Laroque, Pierre, ed. 1962. *Politique de la Viellesse.* Paris: Docum. Francaise.

Lion, Robert, ed. 1980. *Vieillir Demain.* Paris: Docum. Française.

Montaigne, Michel de. 1595. *Essais,* 3rd ed., Book III, Chapter XIII, Translated by Donald Frame. Los Angeles: Stanford University Press.

Muhlbock, O. 1957. "The Use of Inbred Strains of Animals in Experimental Gerontology." In *Methodology of the Study of Aging,* edited by G.E.W. Wolstenholme and C.M. O'Connor, pp. 115–25. London: J. and A. Churchill.

Myerhoff, Barbara. 1979. *Number Our Days.* New York: E.P. Dutton.

Plato. "Apologia" from *The Republic,* translated by Benjamin Jowett.

Proust, Marcel. 1927. *Le temps retrouvé,* translated by A. Mayor. London: Chatto and Windus.

Ricoeur, Paul. 1971. "The Model of the Text: Meaningful Action Considered as a Text." *Social Research* 38:529–62.

Ricoeur, Paul. 1950. *Freedom and Nature: The Voluntary and the Involuntary.* Translated by E.V. Kohak. Chicago: Northwestern University Press.

Riegel, Klaus. 1973. "On the History of Psychological Gerontology." In *The Psychology of Adult Development and Aging,* edited by Carl Eisdorfer and M. Powell Lawton, pp. 37–68. Washington, D.C.: American Psychological Association.

Schaie, K. Warner. 1973. "Developmental Processes and Aging." In *The Psychology of Adult Development and Aging,* edited by Carl Eisdorfer and M. Powell Lawton, pp. 151–56. Washington, D.C.: American Psychological Association.

Shock, Nathan, ed. 1960. *Aging: Some Social and Biological Aspects.* Washington, D.C.: American Association for the Advancement of Science.

Taylor, Charles. 1971. "Interpretation and the Sciences of Man." *The Review of Metaphysics* 25:3–51.

United Nations. 1980. *Report of the General Secretary: Problems of the Elderly and the Aged.* New York: United Nations Organization.

13 CULTURAL INFLUENCES ON AGING

Erdman Palmore

Cultural factors are of critical importance in understanding aging and the aged in any society. Indeed, the very definition of who is considered "elderly" is determined by the culture, which varies from society to society. In some preliterate societies the elderly are not defined by chronological age, but by some achieved status such as becoming a grandparent, or becoming head of a clan, or being appointed to a council of elders. Other societies define the elderly as those who are no longer physically or mentally competent to carry out normal activities. Most Western societies, in contrast, define the elderly as those over age sixty-five, regardless of achieved status or competence.

Age sixty-five, is of course , a completely arbitrary age that was first picked by Chancellor Bismarck of Germany in 1883 to define the elderly for social security purposes. Bismarck wanted to start giving social security benefits to some elderly in order to weaken the appeal of socialism, but he did not want the program to cost too much, so he picked age sixty-five because few Germans survived much beyond that age in 1883. Today in Germany (East and West) about 15 percent of the population is sixty-five or older. In the United States today 11 percent are sixty-five or over, and this will probably increase

257

to 12 percent by the end of the century. There are serious proposals to raise the age of eligibility for retirement benefits to sixty-eight or even seventy. These proposals are getting widespread support because of the ever-increasing life expectancy and potential productivity of older Americans, as well as the ever-increasing cost of retirement benefits to all at age sixty-five.

Attitudes toward and treatment of elders vary widely from society to society—from gerontocracies where elders run the society, and ancestor worshipping societies such as traditional Japan where elders are honored and given precedence because of their age, to the United States where there is widespread prejudice and discrimination against elders. Many people are so impressed by the obvious physical deterioration and intellectual slowing that usually result from aging that they overlook the central role of culture and society in determining individual and group variations in the aging process. Many differences between younger and older persons are mistakenly attributed to biological aging. For example, the fact that a majority of Japanese men past age sixty-five continue to work while less than a third in the United States do is explained by cultural differences, not biological differences. Similarly, the fact that three-fourths of women over sixty-five in India and Algeria are widows, while only one-third of such women in Haiti and Dominican Republic are widows, is caused by cultural differences, not biological differences, between these countries.

In many developing countries, most of the care and support of elders is provided by their families; however, in developed countries, most of this care and support is provided by government and private agencies. All developed countries spend large sums of money for the care and treatment of elders, with little understanding of the cultural and social factors in aging. As a result, much of this money is wasted: the care is often too little or too late, but sometimes it is too much and too early.

Many people believe that the aged inevitably suffer a steady deterioration in physical and mental abilities and therefore should withdraw from the mainstream of our society. We often forget that in other cultures the aged are the most powerful, the most engaged, and the most respected members of the society. When some aged show depression, hopelessness, inferiority feelings, paranoia, and psychosomatic symptoms, we often forget that they may have been caused by deprivation, role loss, status loss, and discrimination rather than by any biological process. Indeed, the noted biologist and gerontologist Alex Comfort estimates that only one-quarter of age-related changes are accounted for by physical aging. The other three-fourths are accounted for by "sociogenic aging, the role which our folk-lore, our prejudices, and our misconceptions about age still impose on the old" (Comfort 1977).

In order to illustrate these cultural influences on aging, we will first examine the main cultural prejudices and discriminations against elders in our society, then take an overview of modernization and aging, with specific attention to the exceptional case of Japan, and close with a look at cultural influences on gerontology.

PREJUDICES[1]

Just as racial groups suffer from racism and women suffer from sexism, the aged in our society suffer from ageism— prejudice and discrimination against the aged. Because ageism is a relatively new concept and is so much a part of our culture, much of it tends to be unrecognized and unconscious, but it is none the less real and damaging to the health and happiness of our elders.

Illness

One of the most common prejudices in our culture is that most older people are ill or disabled. From one-fifth to two-thirds of various groups agree with the following statements: Older people "spend much time in bed because of illness"; "have many accidents in the home"; "have poor coordination"; "feel tired most of the time"; and "develop infection easily" (Tuckman and Lorge 1958). Other common stereotypes are that large proportions of the aged are living in hospitals, nursing homes, homes

1. Some of this material is based on Palmore 1980a.

for the aged, or other such institutions, and that the health and abilities of the aged show a steady decline with each passing year (Palmore 1977).

The fact is that these stereotypes do not apply to the vast majority of elders. For instance, it comes as a great surprise to those unfamiliar with the facts that only 5 percent of persons aged sixty-five and over live in homes for the aged, nursing homes, hospitals, or other institutions (U.S. Census 1970). In an ordinary group of uninformed persons, estimates of the proportion of aged who live in institutions usually range from 20 percent to over 50 percent.

As for the idea that the aged spend much time in bed due to illness, it is true that they spend almost twice as many days in bed per year as younger persons, but this is still only 3 percent of the total days in the year (ten days for men, thirteen days for women) (National Center for Health Statistics 1977). Also, most aged persons are able to perform their major activity most of the time. Only 16 percent of the aged outside institutions say that they are unable to perform their major activity. The average number of restricted activity days is only thirty-eight per year.

In reference to the stereotype that the aged develop infections easily and have many accidents, there are actually fewer acute conditions among the old than among the young (1.1 per person per year for the aged compared to 2.3 for persons under age sixty-five). It is true that the elderly have more chronic conditions (81 percent), but this is only one and one-half times more than those aged seventeen to sixty-four (54 percent) and includes such minor conditions as a need for glasses, mild hearing loss, and allergies.

Regarding the belief that the health and physical ability of most aged persons decline steadily, the Duke Longitudinal Study of Aging found that from 44 percent to 58 percent of survivors who returned for examinations had no decline in physical functioning or actually had some improvement over time, depending on the time interval (three to thirteen years) (Palmore 1970). The aged actually show great variability in patterns of change. A few decline precipitously and quickly become totally disabled. For the majority of aged, however, health and abilities seem to remain fairly level or fluctuate slightly when illnesses are contracted, accidents occur, and recoveries are made; 51 percent of the aged rate their health as good, 33 percent as fair, and only 16 percent as poor (Epstein 1967). Some aged pride themselves on remaining extremely healthy and capable. There are frequent reports of older persons who run marathons, climb mountains, swim great distances, and carry out other feats demonstrating their high level of physical functioning. One study reports that a one-year program of exercise for men seventy and over so improved their health and fitness that their body reactions became similar to those of men thirty years younger (Devries 1968). Such evidence suggests that much of the decline in abilities that does occur among the aged may be due more to declining exercise and activity than to any inevitable aging process itself. In most developing countries, it is assumed that most elders will remain healthy enough to continue normal activities until shortly before death.

Impotency

A related prejudice against the aged is the belief that most no longer have any sexual activity or even sexual desire, and that those few who do are morally perverse or at least abnormal. Evidence from surveys shows these beliefs to be false. The Duke Longitudinal Study of Aging indicates that large proportions of the elderly continue to be sexually active, with even larger proportions reporting continuing interest in sexual activity. For example, 70 percent of the men who were relatively healthy reported that they were still sexually active, and 80 percent reported continuing sexual interest (Palmore 1970). Sexual activity and interest did tend to decline with advancing age, but the majority of men continued to be sexually active up through their seventies.

This bias against sexual activity among the aged often causes resistance to remarriage and other normal sexual interests. Clinicians should be aware that frustration of sexual desire among the aged, as at any age, may cause depression and other psychiatric symptoms. Many other cultures not only assume most older couples will remain sexually active, but also believe such activity contributes to health and happiness.

Mental Decline

Another common belief is that mental abilities begin to decline steadily from age twenty onward, especially the abilities to learn and remember, so that "you can't teach an old dog new tricks," and the aged are generally mentally incompetent. It is true that reaction time tends to slow somewhat with advancing age, but among healthy aged this slowing is only about two-tenths of a second on the average and has little practical significance for most tasks and functioning (Palmore 1970). Furthermore, there is great variability in reaction times, and many older persons have faster reaction times than the average young person. It is also true that older persons often require somewhat longer to learn new material, but given extra time, they can learn as well as younger persons.

As for general intelligence, longitudinal studies found little or no overall decline with age among the healthy aged until a few years before death. Tests of vocabulary and information also show less decline than performance tests involving speed response. Similarly, there tends to be a decline in speed of response but not in accuracy. Seven different studies have found that subjects with advanced education and superior ability, working without time pressure, show little or no deterioration with age (Palmore 1974). In many other cultures, it is assumed that one's mental abilities increase with age and experience. The "wise men" of the society are usually the older men.

Mental Illness

A similar prejudice is that many or most aged are "senile" and that mental illness is common, inevitable, and untreatable among most older people. This view is particularly vicious because it can become a self-fulfilling prophecy in which the belief that mental illness is inevitable and untreatable leads to lack of prevention and treatment, which in turn tends to confirm the original belief.

The facts clearly contradict such beliefs. Less than 1 percent of persons over sixty-five are patients in mental hospitals. An additional 1 percent or 2 percent have significant psychiatric disturbances and reside in other institutions (Redick et al. 1973). As for those living outside institutions, a series of eight community surveys found the prevalence of psychosis to vary from 4 percent to 8 percent (Riley and Foner 1968). All the studies agree that severe mental illness is not inevitable for the majority of older persons, even with the current levels of social and psychological stress in our society. The prevalence of milder forms of mental illness becomes largely a matter of arbitrary definition, and the estimates of psychoneurosis range from 7 percent to over 50 percent, but these are not much larger than for the total population.

Uselessness

Because of these widespread beliefs that the majority of the aged are disabled by physical or mental illness, many people conclude that the elderly are unable to continue working and that those few who do continue to work are unproductive. It is true that, in this country, the majority of the aged are retired, but evidence indicates that this is due less to disability than to discrimination in employment (such as compulsory retirement) and other pressures for the aged to withdraw from the labor force (Palmore 1972). In such countries as Japan, older workers are highly valued, and the majority continue to work past age sixty-five (Palmore 1975). Even in this country, most persons over sixty-five either continue to be employed (12 percent), continue to work as homemakers (17 percent), do volunteer work (another 19 percent), or are retired but would like to be employed or do volunteer work (30 percent). Thus, a total of 78 percent are working (including housework and volunteer work) or would like to have some kind of work (Harris 1975).

Isolation

The idea that most aged are lonely and isolated from their families and normal social relations is clearly false. About 80 percent of the aged in the United States live with someone else, 75 percent say they are not often alone, and 86 percent say they have seen one or more relatives during the previous week (Shanas 1968). Two studies also found that there is even more social interaction and less isolation among aged who live in neighborhoods with a high proportion of other aged persons (Rosenberg 1968; Rosow 1967). About two-thirds say they are never, or hardly ever, lonely, or say that loneliness is not a serious problem (Harris 1975). Most older persons have close relatives within easy visiting distance, and contacts are relatively frequent (Binstock and Shanas 1976). About one-half of the aged say they "spend a lot of time" socializing with friends. Three-fourths are members of a church or synagogue (Erskine 1964), and about half attend services at least three times per month (Hausknecht 1962). Over half belong to other voluntary organizations. Thus, between visits with relatives and friends and participation in church and other voluntary organizations, the majority of old people are far from socially isolated. However, when isolation and loneliness do occur, they may contribute to mental illness, especially depression and cognitive disorientation. In non-Western societies, the aged are even less isolated.

Poverty

Views about the economic status of the aged range from those who think that most of the aged live in poverty, to those who think that a large proportion of the aged are rich with substantial assets. Neither of these extreme views is correct. It is true that the average income of older persons is cut approximately in half after retirement and about 15 percent of persons over sixty-five have incomes below the poverty level according to the official government definitions (Fowles 1977). But this is only 3 percent more than for those under age sixty-five. Our elders have as high or higher standards of living than elders in most other countries.

DISCRIMINATION

Employment

Perhaps the most obvious and serious form of discrimination is in the area of employment: from hiring and promotions to firing and compulsory retirement. Despite the existence of the Age Discrimination in Employment Act, which has been extended to protect workers up to age seventy from discrimination, there is considerable evidence that widespread discrimination against older workers persists (Binstock and Shanas 1976). Compulsory retirement based on age is by definition discrimination against an age category. Compulsory retirement is a policy that prevents employment of older persons regardless of their personal merit, abilities, or qualifications.

Contrary to our prejudices against older workers, the facts indicate that most older workers can work at least as effectively as younger workers. Despite declines in perception and reaction speed under laboratory conditions among the general aged population, studies of older workers under actual working conditions generally show that they perform as well as young workers, if not better on most measures. When speed of reaction is important, older workers usually produce at lower rates, but they are at least as accurate and steady in their work as younger workers. Consistency of output tends to increase with age, as older workers perform at steadier rates from week to week than younger workers do. In addition, older workers have less job turnover, less stress, fewer accidents, less absenteeism, and more job satisfaction than younger workers (Rosow and Zager 1980).

The evidence does not justify age discrimination on most jobs. In fact, such discrimination often results in such detrimental effects as loss of income, loss of role and status, isolation, depression, and declining health and vigor because of inactivity. Unlike ours, many other societies assume that ability on the job does not decline with age, and they value older, experienced workers more than younger ones (Palmore 1975).

Inadequate Medical Care

It is difficult to assess the adequacy of medical care for elders. On the one hand, elders are the only age group covered by national health insurance (Medicare), and they certainly consume a larger proportion of health services than any other group. On the other hand, there are several indications that they still receive less adequate care than other age groups. First, the widespread belief (often shared by the aged themselves) that most of the illnesses and health conditions of older persons are normal and irreversible, prevents the adequate treatment of many illnesses that are in fact reversible. This is an example of a self-fulfilling prophecy, in that the belief that something is untreatable leads to neglect, which may eventually make the condition untreatable. Second, there is extensive evidence that most health professionals tend to give low priority to treating the aged and prefer to treat children and young adults (Palmore 1977). Third, despite Medicare, there are still formidable barriers to adequate care, including financial and transportation barriers as well as ignorance and denial among elders. Fourth, despite the fact that elders consume more health services, these moderately higher rates of consumption are still lower than might be expected based on the much higher rates of illness and health concerns among older people. It is probable that many elders do not get as adequate medical care as they would if they were younger. In most socialist countries health care is free, and even in most nonsocialist countries, health care is less expensive for elders than in the United States.

Other Discrimination

There are many other areas where subtle and sometimes not-so-subtle discrimination against elders is practiced. The aged sometimes have more difficulty getting a loan or mortgage, even though their life expectancy would cover the period of payments on the loan. They are usually not given the educational opportunities younger persons have. Civic and community organizations often drop them out of active leadership roles. Commercials and advertisements depicting older persons usually show them as suffering from arthritis, constipation, insomnia, or some other ailment. Slang epithets for older persons are widely used: dirty old man, old geezer, old codger, old maid, old biddy, old bag, hag, senile, and decrepit. Most jokes and sayings about the aged tend to reinforce prejudice against them (Palmore 1971). Even supposed compliments such as "You don't look that old" and "You haven't changed a bit" imply that to look old or older is to look ugly or infirm.

As a result of these prejudices and discriminations, most older persons tend to deny their age and suffer from lowered self-esteem when they have to admit their age. Some stop having birthdays; others give their age as "thirty-nine" for the rest of their lives. One of the most common types of jokes about the aged involves denial of age. In normal conversation with elders it is considered rude and embarrassing to ask about or discuss the elder's age. If the age is revealed, the older person is usually reassured that "You don't look that old." Billions of dollars are spent each year in such attempts to hide signs of aging as hair dyes, toupees, hair growers, wrinkle removers, and face lifts. The elderly should not be criticized for these attempts to look "handsome" or "beautiful," yet these attempts only demonstrate our basic assumption that youth is beautiful and desirable, while old age is ugly and undesirable.

In contrast, many cultures in less industrialized countries and in Asia still admire and venerate old age. Gray hair, baldness, and wrinkles tend to be respected as badges of maturity, experience, wisdom, and service. In Japan, for example, it is generally considered respectful to ask an elder's age and then to congratulate the elder on this advanced age and venerability (Palmore 1975).

MODERNIZATION AND THE AGED

How did these prejudices and discriminations come about? One clue is that they are largely confined to some modern societies, particularly Western societies, and most especially to the United States.

When we compare the status of the aged in different cultures around the world and in different societies throughout history, a pattern begins to emerge. This pattern could be represented by a curvilinear graph of the rise and fall in status of the aged in the following general form. The baseline or zero point would be represented by animal groups in which there seem to be no instincts or inborn propensities to sustain aged parents or grandparents. The usual pattern among animals is to abandon the aged of the species as soon as their ability to function has seriously declined (Simmons 1960). It is only through the development of human culture that the aged have been able to achieve any security. Beginning with primitive hunting, fishing, and collecting societies, the status and security of the aged rises until it reaches its peak in highly developed argricultural societies. Simmons and others have argued that the graph would show substantial decline as it moves to our modern industrial societies (Cowgill and Holmes 1972).

The reasons for the rise in status of the aged from the primitive to the stable rural societies involve six factors that may be summarized as follows:

1. Stable agricultural societies were able to develop greater surpluses of food and shelter with the aged.
2. Stable agricultural societies developed more capital and more personal property, which increasingly came under the control of the aged.
3. The growing importance of extended family relations could also be manipulated by the aged to support their status and power.
4. In agricultural societies there are generally more opportunities for auxiliary but useful tasks for the aged than in the more primitive ones.

5. Stable agrarian societies accumulated more and more knowledge and technical skills for adapting to the environment and meeting the needs of its members. The aged tended to be the best authorities on this accumulated knowledge and often the most skilled practitioners of the growing arts and crafts.

6. Similarly, because of their greater experience and knowledge, the aged were usually able to become the main leaders in the growing political, civil, judicial, and religious institutions in the agrarian society. These roles were even more rewarding than their auxiliary tasks. Simmons found that most of the tribes he surveyed had old men as chiefs, councilmen, and advisors. He pointed out that the term "elder" had commonly implied leader, head man, or councilman. Also, as magic and religion were associated with complex ceremonies and institutions among the sedentary societies, the aged were usually able to control the most important roles in these structures.

This general picture of the high status given the aged in agricultural societies needs two qualifications, however. First, the aged in some foraging, hunting, and fishing societies had relatively high status, and the aged in some agricultural societies had relatively low status (Friedman 1960). Second, among all societies, the extremely old and helpless person is viewed as a living liability (Simmons 1960).

There seems to be little question that the status of the aged in most stable agricultural societies tended to be higher than in most primitive societies. However, the assumption that the status and satisfactions of the aged have declined markedly as a result of industrialization is more debatable. Shanas (1968), Friedman (1960), and others have challenged the view that today's aged are less socially integrated and are worse off than the aged were a century ago.

Several distinctions need to be made in resolving this issue. First, the different types of status or satisfaction need to be specified (e.g., health, economic, family, political, prestige). For example, there is evidence that the health, education, and income status of the aged as a group are improving as younger and healthier cohorts move into the aged category and as health care improves (Palmore 1976). Also, the actual standard of living of the aged has probably improved over the past century, just as it has for the average younger person. On the other hand, the proportion of the aged living with children or other relatives has declined (Golant 1975), although the extended kinship network remains strong (Shanas 1968).

The status of the aged relative to younger people has probably declined in several industrial societies, although this decline may be leveling off or even reversing itself in the most advanced nations like the United States and Canada (Palmore and Manton 1974).

Finally, trends in the status of the aged vary substantially by race, sex, and socioeconomic status. Therefore it is neither useful nor accurate to make such a broad generalization as "the status of the aged declines as a result of industrialization." Accurate resolution of the issue requires specification of the country, the kind of status meant, how status is measured, and which type of aged person is being referred to.

ORIENTAL SOCIETIES

The status of the aged in the Asian societies appears to have suffered much less decline than in the Western societies. For example, aging in Japan is almost the opposite of aging in the United States. Despite high levels of industrialization and urbanization, the Japanese have maintained a high level of respect for their elders and a high level of integration of their elders in the family, work force, and community. Old age is recognized by most Japanese as a source of prestige and honor. The most common word for the aged in Japanese, *Otoshiyori*, literally means "the honorable elders." Respect for the elders is shown in the honorific language used in speaking to or about them; rules of etiquette which give precedence to the elders in seating arrangements, serving order, bathing order, and going through doors; bowing to the elders; the national holiday called Respect for Elders Day; giving seats on crowded public vehicles to the elders; and the authority of the elders over many family and household matters.

The high level of their integration into Japanese society is demonstrated by the following facts. Over 75 percent of all Japanese aged sixty-five and older live with their children, in contrast to 25 percent in the United States. The majority of Japanese men over sixty-five continue to serve in the labor force, compared to 29 percent of men in the United States over sixty-five. Most of the Japanese elders who are not actually employed continue to be useful in housekeeping, child care, shopping, and gardening, often freeing their daughters or daughters-in-law for employment outside the home. The vast majority of Japanese elders also remain active in their communities through senior citizens clubs, religious organizations, and informal neighborhood groups. Most surprising of all, there appears to have been relatively little decline in these high levels of integration during the past twenty or thirty years.

This high status of elders in Japan is rooted in two cultural traditions: filial piety and a vertical social structure. Filial piety, or support and honor for parents and grandparents, comes in turn from two religious traditions: ancestor worship and Confucianism. Traditional Japanese worshiped their ancestors because they believed that upon death, their ancestors' spirits became the controlling forces in their lives. Thus it was important to please and placate their ancestors, both living and dead, in order to have a good life. The Confucian tradition is based on respect for parental authority in the home and civil authority outside the home. One of the highest virtues in Confucianism is filial piety. The vertical social structure makes the important people in your life those who are above or below you—parents and children, bosses and subordinates—in contrast to our more horizontal structure, where the more important people are those on a level with you—siblings, fellow workers, and peers.

Observers in the Peoples' Republic of China and in Taiwan also report relatively high status for the aged (Cowgill and Holmes 1972). Thus, Asian societies prove that the aged in industrial societies need not suffer from the ageism they experience in our society.

CULTURAL INFLUENCES ON GERONTOLOGY

Countries can be grouped into five categories or stages in terms of their development of gerontology (Cowgill 1980). In the first stage there is no gerontology of any form: no research, no teaching, and usually no specialized service programs. These are the developing societies (e.g., Brazil, Peru, Iran, Jordan, Nigeria, and American Samoa) in which demographic aging has not yet occurred to any measurable degree, and in which older persons are cared for and integrated into familial and kinship systems. All of them have less than 3 percent of their population over age sixty-five. Their present social problems are overwhelmingly concerned with youth.

However, in several other countries with no greater proportions of aged, there are indications of stage two: some beginning interest in research relative to aging. In each case this is either a transplanted interest stimulated by contact with gerontology elsewhere or a response to some specific problem. Countries that presently typify stage two are Thailand, Egypt, Taiwan, Kuwait, and Kenya.

The third stage is to be found in such places as Australia and Japan where we have both biomedical and sociological research, much of which is taking place within organized structures such as institutes on aging, and is being published in scientific journals. There are still almost no formal courses in gerontology, and few faculty members describe themselves as gerontologists. In these societies about 7 or 8 percent of the population is age sixty-five or over, and this proportion is increasing rapidly.

The fourth stage is represented by societies which have developed a full range of academic programs in gerontology, including not only research institutes, associations, and journals, but also formal courses and faculty who identify themselves as gerontologists both for research and teaching. Many of the countries in Western Europe are in stage four: Sweden, Austria, West Germany, Holland, and France. All of these countries have populations with 14 or 15 percent of the population age sixty-five and over. Israel is also in this stage, with only 9 percent age sixty-five and over, but a large proportion are migrants from Europe who have developed programs on the European model. Canada is also in this stage with only 8 percent of its people age sixty-five and over, but is influenced by its neighbor the United States.

The fifth stage is reached when the national government formally sponsors gerontological research and training. The United States is the clearest example of this stage, but Norway and the United Kingdom are entering it. Several other countries will probably move into this stage soon.

In all countries, until recently most gerontology has been limited in two ways: it has tended to be negative and to be provincial. It has been negative in emphasizing the problematic aspects of aging rather than the advantages and opportunities of normal aging. There are many reasons for this. As the proportion of aged in a country increases rapidly, people become alarmed at the burden of supporting and caring for so many dependent people. It is also easier to study "captive" groups of aged in clinics, hospitals, and nursing homes, forgetting that these groups represent only 5 or 10 percent of the total aged population. In addition, the motivation for research is often to convince decisionmakers that something needs to be done. As a result, there has been an emphasis on counting the problem cases and a tendency to exaggerate the seriousness of the problem. Much of the research prior to the last decade was of this kind, and it tended to reinforce the prejudices reviewed here. It is more difficult and costly to study a normal representative sample over a long enough period of time to see the real consequences of aging. Only recently in stages four and five has gerontology revised its methods and interpretations to provide a more balanced view of the negatives and positives in normal aging.

The other limitation—provincialism—has resulted from the concentration of most gerontologists on aging in their country alone. Cross-cultural gerontology has been rare, and most gerontology has been limited to the United States and a few Western European countries: consequently, most of what we knew about aging is derived from data on white populations in Western, capitalist countries (Palmore 1980). Yet we need to expand our views of aging among other races, cultures, and economic and political systems. It is only through such cross-cultural studies that gerontology will become a truly international science and profession; and only by taking a world perspective will we overcome our provincialism and develop a more universal understanding of aging. And after all, aging is that culminating stage of life to which we all aspire.

REFERENCES

Binstock, R., and E. Shanas. 1976. *Handbook of Aging and the Social Sciences*. New York: Van Nostrand Reinhold.
Comfort, A. 1976. "Real and Imaginary Aging." In *Proceedings: Governor's Conference on the Quality of Life for Our Senior Citizens*. Raleigh: North Carolina Department of Human Resources.
Cowgill, D. 1980. "The International Development of Academic Gerontology." In *International Handbook on Aging*, edited by E. Palmore, pp. 501–06. Westport, Conn.: Greenwood Press.
Cowgill, D., and L. Holmes, eds. 1972. *Aging and Modernization*. New York: Appleton-Century-Crofts.
Devries, H. 1968. *Reports on Jogging and Exercise for Older Adults*. Washington, D.C.: Administration on Aging.
Epstein, L. 1967. *The Aged Population of the U.S.* Washington, D.C.: Government Printing Office.
Erkskine, H. 1964. "The Polls." *Public Opinion Quarterly* 28:679.
Fowles, D. 1977. *Income and Poverty Among the Elderly*. Washington, D.C.: Administration on Aging.
Friedman, D. 1960. "The Impact of Aging on the Social Structure." In *Handbook of Social Gerontology*, edited by C. Tibbets, pp. 120–44. Chicago: University of Chicago Press.
Golant, S. 1975. "Residential Concentrations of the Future Elderly." *Gerontologist* 15:16.
Harris, L. 1975. *The Myth and Reality of Aging in America*. Washington, D.C.: National Council on the Aging.
Hausknecht. M. 1962. *The Joiners*. New York: Bedminister Press.
National Center for Health Statistics. 1977. *National Health Survey*, Series 10. Washington, D.C.: Government Printing Office.
Palmore, E. 1970. *Normal Aging*. Durham: Duke University Press.
Palmore, E. 1971. "Attitudes toward Aging as Shown by Humor." *Gerontologist* 11:181.
Palmore, E. 1972. "Compulsory vs. Flexible Retirement." *Gerontologist* 12:343.
Palmore, E. 1974. *Normal Aging*, vol. II. Durham: Duke University Press.

Palmore, E. 1975. *The Honorable Elders*. Durham: Duke University Press.

Palmore, E. 1976. "The Future Status of the Aged." *Gerontologist* 16:297.

Palmore, E. 1977. "Facts on Aging: A Short Quiz." *Gerontologist* 17:315.

Palmore, E. 1979. "The Advantages of Aging." *Gerontologist* 19:220.

Palmore, E. 1980a. "The Social Factors in Aging." In *Handbook of Geriatric Psychiatry*, edited by E. Busse and D. Blazer, pp. 222–48. New York: Van Nostrand Reinhold.

Palmore, E. 1980b. *International Handbook on Aging*. Westport, Conn.: Greenwood Press.

Redick, R., et al. 1973. "Epidemiology of Mental Illness and Utilization of Psychiatric Facilities among Older Persons." In *Mental Illness in Later Life*, edited by E. Busse and E. Pfeiffer, pp. 199–232. Washington, D.C.: American Psychiatric Association.

Riley, M., and A. Foner. 1968. *Aging and Society*, vol. I. New York: Russel Sage Foundation.

Rosenberg, G. 1968. "Age, Poverty, and Isolation from Friends in the Urban Working Class." *Journal of Gerontology* 23:533.

Rosow, L. 1967. *Social Integration of the Aged*. New York: The Free Press.

Roscow, J., and R. Zager. 1980. *The Future of Older Workers in America*. Scarsdale: Work in America Institute.

Shanas, E. 1968. *Old People in Three Industrial Societies*. New York: Atherton Press.

Simmons, L. 1960. "Aging in Preindustrial Societies." In *Handbook of Social Gerontology*, edited by C. Tibbets, pp. 62–91. Chicago: University of Chicago Press.

Tuckman, J., and I. Lorge. 1958. "The Projection of Personal Symptoms into Stereotypes about Aging." *Journal of Gerontology* 13:70.

U.S. Census. 1970. *Inmates of Institutions*. Washington, D.C.: Government Printing Office.

14 SOCIAL POLICIES AND AGING
A Global Perspective
Walter M. Beattie, Jr.

Gerontologists have long held that the study of human aging requires an interdisciplinary approach and a multidimensional perspective. Physiological and psychosocial information are not enough: it is also essential to have knowledge of the historical, cultural, and environmental contexts in which aging takes place. To present a global perspective on social policies and aging is therefore not possible without a broad overview of the major world trends and issues which form both the contexts for aging and the arenas in which social policies are formulated. Ultimately these trends and issues offer both constraints and possibilities for the realization of global policies.

Looking toward the year 2000, most analysts see current trends toward economic inequality, overpopulation, shortages of resources, and ecological damage reaching a crisis point. In 1980, for example, Robert McNamara warned that third- and fourth-world countries may find themselves in a disastrous economic plight within twenty years; that "despite advances of the last quarter-century, 600 million people are likely to be living in absolute poverty by the year 2000." It is these poorest developing countries where, said Mr. McNamara, "the current global economic situation has imposed particularly severe penalties, a situation they neither caused nor can do much to influence."

It would be tempting to view such an assessment as overly pessimistic. However, the recently published *Global 2000 Report to the President* (Council on Environmental Quality and the Department of State 1980) projects a crisis situation in three other areas—population, natural resources, and the environment—that carries an urgency equal to Mr. McNamara's vision of economic distress. The compilers of the study see

> the potential for global problems of alarming proportions by the year 2000. Environmental, resource and population stresses are intensifying and will increasingly determine the quality of human life on our planet. These stresses are already severe enough to deny many millions of people basic needs for food, shelter, health and jobs, or any hope for betterment. At the same time, the earth's carrying capacity—the ability of biological systems to provide resources for human needs—is eroding. The trends . . . suggest strongly a progressive degradation and impoverishment of the earth's natural resource base (p. iii).

The *Global Report* has as one of its major foci "the probable changes in the world's population," yet it does not identify or speak to the aging of the world's population, even though its population projections assume that "life expectancies at birth for the world will increase 11 percent, for the 1975–2000 period, to 65.5 years."

A closer look at global population growth is provided by Rafael Salas, executive director of the United Nations Fund For Population Activities. In his *1979 Report* on the fund's work, Mr. Salas notes:

> During the remaining two decades of this century, close to 2 billion would be added to the world population and this would be almost equal to what was added between 1950 and 1980. Over 90 percent of this increase will occur in the less developed countries and their population alone by the year 2000 would be nearly twice the total population the world had in 1950. By the year 2000, 80 percent of the world population would be living in the less developed countries.

Salas also projects an increase in the rates of migration of population, a particularly unsettling trend for the United

States, where "for the period 1970–1974, 70 percent of the total immigrants . . . came from the less developed countries." The high rates of immigration from Latin America, particularly Mexico, the Caribbean, and South Asia suggest a new kind of aging American, no longer drawn mainly from the developed countries of Europe. They will not only bring far different social and cultural identities and expectations to their old age, but will also bring high levels of illiteracy in the dominant language unless access to lifelong learning becomes a right of all our residents.

However, such large increases in population and migration will put particular pressure on developing countries. As Salas points out, "the less developed countries often lack technical administrative and managerial resources. The bulk of their labor force constitutes unskilled labour and their productivity is also affected by factors such as malnutrition, poor health, inadequate health care and lack of educational facilities." Adequate health care has particular impact upon aging in such countries. As Salas points out:

> Life expectancy figures provide a good summary measure of the status of the health of a population. Life expectancy in 1975–80 was only 54 years for the less developed countries compared to 68 years for the more developed countries. Life expectancy figures reflect mortality rates and an increase in life expectancy is, therefore, closely linked to the expansion of health care facilities and to improvement of nutritional levels.

The role of education in the development of human resources is another broad policy concern. Estimates of illiteracy provided by UNESCO show that in most of Africa more than 50 percent of the population over the age of fifteen were illiterate in 1980. The same is true for South Asia and the Middle East. There are also a few countries in Africa, South Asia, and the Middle East where the proportion of illiterates in the total population is over 90 percent. It can be assumed that an even larger proportion of illiteracy will be found among the aged than for the population as a whole in such regions.

It is against the background of these sobering trends that the increase in aged in the world's population should be noted. Between the years 1970 and 2000 all age groups are expected to increase by 73 percent; the population age sixty and over will increase by 91 percent while the eighty-and-over population will increase by 119 percent, almost half again as rapidly as the world's population of all ages. Nonetheless few, if any, assessments of global trends for the purpose of social policy formulation and planning take into account the fact that mortality has been progressively postponed throughout the world; nor do they consider the impact of aging on institutional arrangements and resource mobilization and allocation.

At the same time, if we are to identify issues for policy formulation and planning, and if we are to develop new institutional responses to the world's aging population, we must concern ourselves with the aggregate numbers as well as the proportions of older persons compared to other age groups (Beattie 1978). For example, the fact that the sixty-and-over population has nearly doubled from 304 million to 581 million between 1970 and 2000 has far greater implications than their percentages—8.4 percent and 9.3 percent of the world's total population—would suggest (see Table 14–1).

From Table 14–2, 1970 can be identified as the transition year in the aging of the world's population. The then-estimated 304 million persons aged sixty years and over were almost evenly divided between the more developed and less developed regions. Since then, more older persons are to be found in the

Table 14–1. The Elderly Population of the World (in Thousands) as a Percentage of the World's Total Population and the Percentage Change, 1970–2000.

| Age | 1970 | | 2000 | | |
	Number	Percentage of World's Total	Number	Percentage of World's Total	Percentage Change
60 and over	304,341	8.4	581,431	9.3	+ 91.05
80 and over	26,327	0.7	57,605	0.9	+118.81
All ages	3,610,377	100.0	6,254,377	100.0	+ 73.23

Source: *Population by Sex and Age for Regions and Countries, 1950-2000, as Assessed in 1973: Medium Variant* (UN, ESA/P/WP60, February 25, 1976).

Table 14-2. The Elderly Population (in Thousands) of the World and Its More- and Less-Developed Regions, 1970 and 2000, as Compared to All Ages and the Percentage Distribution between Regions, and the 80-and-Over Age Group as Percentages of the 60-and-Over Population.

Age	World 1970	World 2000	More-Developed Regions 1970	More-Developed Regions 2000	Less-Developed Regions 1970	Less-Developed Regions 2000
All ages	3,610,377	6,254,377	1,084,018	1,360,245	2,526,359	4,894,133
Percentage	100.0	100.0	30.0	21.8	70.0	78.2
60 and over	304,341	581,431	153,424	233,851	150,917	347,579
Percentage	100.0	100.0	50.4	40.3	49.6	59.7
80 and over	26,327	57,605	16,097	31,203	10,230	26,402
Percentage	100.0	100.0	61.1	54.2	38.9	45.8
80 and over as a percentage of 60 and over	8.6	9.9	10.5	13.3	6.8	7.6

Source: *Population by Sex and Age for Regions and Countries, 1950–2000, as Assessed in 1973: Medium Variant* (UN, ESA/P/WP60, February 25, 1976).

less developed regions. By the year 2000, it is projected that these numbers will increase by 130 percent to 347.6 million in the less developed regions and to 233.9 million, or by some 52 percent, in the more developed regions. The majority of today's older persons are living in the third and fourth worlds, and these numbers continue to increase more rapidly than for the more developed industrialized regions of the world. Therefore, one of the fundamental social policy issues in aging is the fact that those areas of the world which are growing more rapidly in population, and which are facing increasingly diminished physical resources—food, water, energy, minerals, agriculture—are also the same regions where the numbers of the world's older persons are increasing the most rapidly.

This is also true for the very old age group, those eighty and over, which numbered some 26 million in 1970 (see Table 14-3). At that time, 61 percent of the very old were found in the more developed regions, and 39 percent in the less developed regions. By the year 2000, however, this older age group will

Table 14–3. The Elderly Population of the World, Its More- and Less-Developed Regions, and Major Regions (in Thousands) by Sex, 1970 and 2000.

| | 1970 | | | | | | 2000 | | | | | |
| | Men | | Women | | Sex | | Men | | Women | | Sex | |
Area	Number	% Men	Number	% Women	Ratio		Number	% Men	Number	% Women	Ratio	
					Age 60 and Over							
World	135,228	44.43	169,113	55.57	79		265,506	45.66	315,925	54.34	84	
More developed	62,543	40.77	90,880	59.23	68		99,490	42.54	134,361	57.46	74	
Less developed	72,685	48.16	78,231	51.84	92		166,015	47.76	181,564	52.24	91	
Africa	7,708	46.14	8,996	53.86	85		19,358	45.94	22,777	54.06	84	
Latin America	7,746	46.99	8,738	53.01	88		19,242	46.34	22,286	53.66	86	
Northern America	13,628	43.58	17,646	56.42	77		17,905	41.67	25,059	58.33	71	
East Asia	36,714	46.87	41,619	53.13	88		75,150	47.63	82,620	52.37	90	
South Asia	27,144	50.27	26,854	49.73	101		66,168	48.14	71,275	51.86	92	
Europe	31,980	41.83	44,470	58.17	71		43,828	43.85	56,120	56.15	78	
Oceania	935	44.93	1,146	55.07	81		1,694	46.65	1,937	58.35	87	
USSR	9,373	32.30	19,645	67.70	47		22,158	39.56	33,849	60.44	65	

					Age 80 and Over					
World	9,571	36.35	16,756	63.65	57	21,387	31.13	36,218	62.87	59
More developed	5,076	31.53	11,021	68.47	46	10,082	32.81	21,121	67.69	47
Less developed	4,495	43.94	5,734	56.06	78	11,305	42.82	15,097	57.18	74
Africa	550	44.57	684	55.43	80	1,104	41.98	1,526	58.02	72
Latin America	509	41.55	716	58.45	71	1,564	40.47	2,301	59.53	67
Northern America	986	27.60	2,586	72.40	38	2,396	34.17	4,616	65.83	51
East Asia	2,192	40.58	3,210	59.42	68	6,046	40.54	8,869	59.46	68
South Asia	1,695	46.80	1,927	53.20	87	3,829	45.16	4,650	54.84	82
Europe	2,767	34.08	5,352	65.92	51	4,435	33.65	8,746	66.35	50
Oceania	83	35.62	150	64.38	55	169	38.58	269	61.42	62
USSR	789	27.02	2,131	72.98	37	1,843	26.01	5,242	73.99	35

Source: *Population by Sex and Age for Regions and Countries, 1950–2000, as Assessed in 1973: Medium Variant* (UN, ESA/P/WP60 February 25, 1976).

also shift in numbers and proportions toward the less developed regions, where it is projected that some 46 percent of the world's eighty-and-over population will be found. This older age group will number some 26 million in the less developed regions by the year 2000—about the same number as were living in the entire world in 1970. It is, then, in the less developed regions where the numbers of older persons are increasing at a faster rate than for the world as a whole, with the very old's rate of increase the greatest—that is, 158 percent between 1970 and 2000, as contrasted to 94 percent for this age group in the more developed world, and 119 percent for the entire world.

One final word is needed about proportions and numbers of older persons from a social policy perspective. In the more developed regions of the world—Northern America, Europe, Oceania, and Japan—we find that the greatest numbers of older persons are in the urban areas and the highest proportions in the more rural areas. However, as we examine the world trends, we find that the greatest numbers of the elderly are in the less developed regions, especially in the more rural areas, although the highest proportions of the elderly are in the more developed regions. It is in these areas where the development of social policies and specialized services for the aging have occurred. In the less developed regions, with their large numbers of younger people, the elderly represent a small proportion of persons, and their needs are not as readily identified. At the same time, their numbers are far greater than in the developed regions. It is therefore to individuals that social policy must address itself, and not to proportions of a particular age group in a society.

All areas of the world are also experiencing, as a correlate of aging, an increasingly higher ratio of women to men, particularly among the more advanced ages (see Table 14–3). In 1970, among all regions of the world, only South Asia had a ratio favoring men in the sixty-and-over population—that is, 101. By the year 2000, however, this ratio is projected to decline to 92 men for every 100 women. This greater survival of women is most pronounced among the eighty-and-over age group. In 1970, it was 57 men to 100 women, with a slightly more favorable ratio of 59 by the year 2000 as mortality rates among men improve slightly. In the United States, mortality rates are beginning to show a decline among the population over age seventy-five, especially women. The sex ratio among the elderly is lowest in the Soviet Union, both in 1970 and as projected for the year 2000. For those aged sixty and over, it was 47 in 1970 and anticipated to rise to 65 by 2000. For the eighty-and-over ages, it was 37 for the earlier 1970 period, with an anticipated decrease to 35 by 2000. Some of the most critical as well as complex social policy issues of aging are related to the older woman in all countries of the world.

If we examine the demographic trends in aging by regions of the world, the social policy implications became more obvious. South Asia, which had the largest number of the world's population in 1970 (1.1 billion), will experience an increase of more than 100 percent by the year 2000 (see Table 14–4). Although the sixty-and-over population was only 4.9 percent in this region in 1970 and will represent only 6.1 percent by the year 2000, in numbers there were nearly 54 million persons aged sixty and over in 1970, with this older age group expected to increase to more than 137 million by the year 2000. It will then represent the largest proportionate increase of the sixty-and-over population for any region of the world—that is, 154.5 percent.

East Asia, the region which ranked second in 1970 in total population, with nearly 927 million persons, is expected to increase to 1.3 billion by the year 2000. For both the years 1970 and 2000, East Asia ranks first in the total number of persons aged sixty and over, with more than 78 million in 1970 and nearly 158 million in the year 2000. This represents an increase of more than 100 percent in the sixty-and-over age group during this thirty-year period. The eighty-and-over population in East Asia, which measured only 0.6 percent of all ages in 1970 and 1 percent in 2000, will increase by 176 percent over this time period. This compares with an increase of nearly 48 percent for all ages during this same period. By the year 2000, East Asia will have the greatest number of persons over age eighty—nearly 15 million, almost 2 million more than the more developed region of Europe.

Latin America and Africa can anticipate the largest proportionate increase in their total populations—that is, 119

Table 14–4. The Elderly Age Groups by Regions of the World, 1970 and 2000.

Region	Age	1970		2000		Percent Change 1970–2000
		Number (thousands)	Percentage of All Ages	Number (thousands)	Percentage of All Ages	
Africa	All ages	351,727	100.0	813,681	100.0	+131.3
	60 and over	16,704	4.7	42,133	5.2	+152.2
	80 and over	1,235	0.35	2,629	0.32	+112.9
Latin America	All ages	283,020	100.0	619,929	100.0	+119.0
	60 and over	16,483	5.8	41,529	6.7	+152.0
	80 and over	1,225	0.43	3,865	0.62	+215.5
Northern America	All ages	226,389	100.0	296,199	100.0	+ 30.8
	60 and over	31,276	13.8	42,965	14.5	+ 37.4
	80 and over	3,573	1.6	7,012	2.4	+ 96.2
East Asia	All ages	926,866	100.0	1,370,061	100.0	+ 47.8
	60 and over	78,331	8.5	157,772	11.5	+101.4
	80 and over	5,401	0.58	14,916	1.1	+176.2

South Asia	All ages	1,101,199	100.0	2,267,266	100.0	+105.9
	60 and over	53,997	4.9	137,445	6.1	+154.5
	80 and over	3,622	0.33	8,479	0.37	+134.1
Europe	All ages	459,085	100.0	539,500	100.0	+ 17.5
	60 and over	76,449	16.7	99,947	18.5	+ 30.7
	80 and over	8,118	1.8	13,181	2.4	+ 62.4
Oceania	All ages	19,323	100.0	32,715	100.0	+ 69.3
	60 and over	2,081	10.8	3,632	11.1	+ 74.5
	80 and over	233	1.2	438	1.3	+ 88.0
USSR	All ages	242,768	100.0	315,027	100.0	+ 29.8
	60 and over	29,018	12.0	56,007	17.8	+ 93.0
	80 and over	2,920	1.2	7,085	2.2	+142.6

Source: *Population by Sex and Age for Regions and Countries, 1950–2000, as Assessed in 1973: Medium Variant* (UN, ESA/P/WP60, February 25, 1976).

percent and 131 percent, respectively. For the period from 1970 to 2000, the populations aged sixty and over will increase by 152 percent in both areas. Latin America, however, can expect the most rapid increase of any region among the very old—that is, 215.5 percent.

Unlike the less developed regions where individual aging (numbers of older persons) is occurring more rapidly, the developed regions—Northern America, Europe, Oceania, and the Soviet Union—are experiencing an acceleration of societal aging (proportions of older persons). In these regions birth rates have declined steadily, except for a short period following World War II, with a higher survival rate of persons into the middle and more advanced stages of life. Europe, which had the highest proportion of older persons of any region in 1970— with 16.7 percent of its total population aged sixty years and over—will experience an increase to 18.5 percent by the year 2000. For the Soviet Union this proportion was 12 percent in 1970 and will represent nearly 18 percent by 2000. For Northern America and Oceania the proportions will increase less rapidly and be somewhat lower by the year 2000. Northern America will grow from an over-sixty population of 13.8 percent in 1970 to 14.5 percent in 2000, while Oceania will grow from 10.8 to 11.1 percent at the turn of the next century. Despite the higher proportions of older persons in these more developed regions, their numbers are far less than in the less developed regions.

Still another frequently used method for analyzing the impact of the elderly within a population is the "concept of dependency" ratio (see Table 14–5), which brings together those under age fifteen and those over sixty-five. However, one may question the demographic labeling of the young and the old as comparable or "dependent" in the same manner. The sixty-five-and-over population represents an extremely wide age range, yet applying the same span of years to younger groups, we would not equate those in their late teens and those in their late forties as belonging to a similar age stage, or sharing similar life identities. The sixty-five-year-old and the eighty-five-year-old are indeed "different," yet many social policies for older people package rights, entitlements, and programs as if they were essentially alike. Dependency, economic

Table 14-5. Demographic Profile of the World and Its More- And Less-Developed Countries, 1965–1970 and 2000

	World		More Developed Countries		Less Developed Countries	
	1965-70	2000	1965-70	2000	1965-70	2000
Birth rate	33.8	25.1	18.6	17.5	40.6	27.4
Death rate	14.0	8.1	9.1	9.6	16.1	7.6
Growth rate	2.0	1.7	1.0	0.8	2.4	2.0
Age Structure	100.0	100.0	100.0	100.0	100.0	100.0
Percentage						
Under 15	37.0	32.9	26.8	24.9	41.4	35.2
15-64	57.8	61.0	63.5	63.7	55.3	60.3
65 and over	5.2	6.1	9.6	11.4	3.3	4.6
Average age (median)	26	29	33	35	23	27
Dependency ratio, (total)	74	64	59	57	81	66
Youth (under 15)	65	54	44	39	75	58
Aged (65 and over)	9	10	15	18	6	8
Percentage surviving to age 15	85.9		95.0		82.0	
Expectation of life at birth	53.1	66.5	70.4	73.2	49.6	65.3
Children ever-born	4.7	3.3	2.7	2.5	5.6	3.5
Average number surviving to age 20	4.0	3.1	2.6	2.4	4.6	3.3

Source: Circa 1965–70 adapted from United Nations, 1971, *The World Population Situation in 1970*, (New York: Department of Economic and Social Affairs, *Population Studies*, no. 49; and, the year 2000 adapted from United Nations, 1976, *World and Regional Population Prospects: Addendum, World Population Prospects Beyond the Year 2000*, in Philip M. Hauser, "Aging and World-wide Population Change," in *Handbook of Aging and the Social Sciences*, R. Binstock and E. Shanas, eds. (New York: Van Nostrand Reinhold Company), pp. 69 and 71. Reprinted with permission.

or otherwise, is not the same for older adults as it is with children. In fact, it is a concept that contributes to the all-too-frequent infantilization of our elders. The real issue is not dependence or independence: it is interdependence—that is, helping older persons to become participants and contribute to human society. Too often, social policies purporting to help and support the aging instead separate the old from their families, through eligibility requirements; from their work places, through retirement; and from the larger community, through environmental barriers or specialized housing.

To return to the dependency ratio concept and its implications for social policy, the Noted French demographer Alfred Sauvy (1979) has cogently pointed out that although the proportion of young dependents will decline and the proportion of the elderly dependents will increase, an error is made by policymakers who

> draw reassuring conclusions from this, saying that the proportion of adults remains the same so that the total cost of the inactive will also remain the same. The error is worthy of note: not only is it somewhat strange to consider the replacement of a young person by an old one as "neutral," but the cost to the community (Social Security and education) is two and a half times as much for the old as for the young.

In addition to these major trends, other complex forces and issues are simultaneously having a profound impact on the lives and identities of older persons worldwide. They are the grist for the mill of social policy, effecting basic changes in the scope and structure of human activities throughout the world. As such, they are essential to a global perspective on social policy and aging.

The first such trend is the scientific and technological revolution, which is giving rise to the knowledge and information explosions of the mid-to-late twentieth century. The implications for educational policy are many and include the emergence of continuous life-span education and a lifelong-learning concept. If knowledge is power, then older persons are displaced from centers of power in a society unless they have continuing access to new and changing knowledge and information. Informational obsolescence soon becomes equated with social obsolescence and displacement. These in turn bring about a sense of displacement in the roles and expectations of older persons, as what they had understood when younger to be their social entitlements in old age can no longer be delivered by the society.

Second, we have vast changes in the very nature and meaning of environments. For those who have grown old without moving from their environment, that environment has changed—in the United States, in Japan, in African societies. Indeed, for countless people, the place of their aging is no longer the familiar place of their developing years.

Third, we are experiencing an acceleration of social change, less in the developed than in the developing world, where it has brought a phenomenal extension of the life-span. In fact, the increased longevity that has taken the developed countries a century to achieve is taking only decades in the developing world: this is what Simon Bergman has called the "telescoping of aging."

Fourth, we are undergoing a period of economic inflation-deflation and are coming to grips with perceived limits to the concept of ever-expanding growth. Both of these factors are intimately related to the worldwide energy crisis that first became recognized in the early 1970s, and both factors have crucial implications for aging. The limits of expansion and growth are of particular importance to social policy formulation in the more developed areas of the world.

The trends and issues considered thus far provide a background for examining several broad and highly interrelated social policy issues. The first of these is the right to work and the right to retire; and the second concerns policies of income security, maintenance, and protection in old age. The latter policy issues should be examined first, because in large measure work-retirement policies are dependent on the income issues of old age.

The first social insurance system began, not in Bismarck's Germany in the late 1880s as is generally thought, but rather in Uruguay in 1838, for federal employees in the Central Administration. Nonetheless, the concept of social security did not develop to any degree among national states until the late nineteenth century. Its most rapid growth and expansion occurred after World War II, continuing until the mid-1970s. From 1949 to 1979, programs of income protection for old age, survivors, and invalidity increased nearly threefold, from 44 national programs to 123 such programs. This increase was due largely to the emergence of sixty new countries between

1959 and 1979. As of 1979, there were only nineteen countries without social security programs—the majority of them in the developing regions of the world. The 1960s and the 1970s brought numerous expanded measures as increased benefit awards, broader coverage, lower retirement age, relaxed retirement tests, extended invalidity pension coverage, extended health care, and the addition of new programs. Such changes have led to higher payroll taxes for both employer and employee, along with increased government funding (U.S. Department of Health and Human Services 1980). For the most part, payroll taxes are the main source of revenue; in some instances, general tax revenues contribute (Ross 1979).

Twelve of the developing countries have a special social security system restricted to public employees only. Indeed, such programs usually begin with the military, civil servants, and teachers—the elite in such countries. By far the most prevalent social security programs related to income protection in old age are social insurance programs; these are currently operating in sixty-nine countries, primarily in the developed world. These are contributory programs by which employers and in most instances, employees, provide for a pension in old age, although a few provide only for a lump-sum payment at retirement. Nine of the more developed countries, such as Norway, Sweden, and Canada, also provide a universal old-age pension—basic guaranteed income. Seventeen developing countries maintain a provident fund system—that is, a contributory employer-employee system providing a lump-sum benefit at retirement, usually made up of contributions plus interest. In addition, a means-tested social assistance program is practiced by four countries, including the United Kingdom, which also has a social insurance program.

Despite the commonalities of such programs, they do vary considerably, according to the values and ideologies of each society. Such values and ideologies guide the formulation of policy goals, as well as define the appropriate means for their attainment: they may therefore define the appropriate role and responsibilities of government, the voluntary sector, the family, and the individual. They also determine the allocative processes of a society—who gets how much of what—and define rights and entitlements to goods and services. For example, the Republic of South Africa's social policy of apartheid—official three-way racial segregation—is reflected in its old-age pension system. This provides less than 60 percent of the white population's benefits to coloreds and Asians, and 28 percent of white benefits to blacks (U.S. Department of Health and Human Services 1980).

The chronological age for eligibility for social security benefits also varies greatly from country to country. To a large degree the eligibility also becomes the modal age for removal from the labor force. The youngest age is forty in the Solomon Islands, followed by fifty-five in Swaziland and Nigeria. Fifty-five is the modal age for women in twenty-eight countries, while sixty is the modal age for men, also in twenty-eight countries. In fact, in many countries the eligibility age is five years less for women than for men, despite the mortality and life-expectancy differences favoring women. The highest age—sixty-seven—is found in Norway and Denmark.

Japan's mandatory retirement age—fifty-five—is the earliest among industrialized nations, although one is not eligible for social security benefits until age sixty. As a result, the large majority, primarily men, work beyond the mandatory retirement age, although they are generally rehired by employers at lower pay and usually in a lower position. Such older workers also receive at retirement a lump-sum pension from their employers providing a de facto extension of retirement age without forcing employers to pay the higher costs of formally extending such an age. In the private employment sector, promotions are based primarily on seniority, and the lump-sum retirement benefits are based on the number of years worked and wages at retirement.

The pressures to raise the retirement age in Japan are strong, especially since it has one of the highest life expectations at birth. Some companies have raised mandatory retirement to age sixty. The majority of companies, however, offer employment to older workers while at the same time avoiding the disadvantages of retaining older persons as permanent employees. This is facilitated by a governmental policy that requires companies with more than one hundred employees to draw up plans for hiring older workers and create "reemployment offices." The government provides subsidies of $360 a year for each older worker reemployed (Kii 1978).

Many countries restrict entitlement to benefits according to length of service as well as chronological age. In addition, forty-eight countries require full retirement, eleven require partial or substantial retirement, while twenty have no such requirements. In fourteen developing countries, the concept of premature aging provides for earlier retirement age with full benefits. Others provide a reduced eligibility age for those who have been engaged in hazardous or special occupations. In several countries, women who have borne more than a prescribed number of children also have a reduced age for eligibility. Many index benefits to keep them related to cost-of-living or wage changes. Several provide a supplement for beneficiaries. The majority provide for a dependent's supplement, usually for a wife and school-age children. Many provide a proportionate increment if retirement is delayed beyond the age of eligibility, and a reduction if the retirement age is less than that provided for.

A social security system is only one component of social policy concerned with old-age income security, protection, and maintenance. Others include private or public pension schemes, savings plans, and earnings based on a continuing right to work. Increasingly these separate schemes are centralized under one administrative mechanism and interrelated around social policy concerns.

One such concern is the question of how much is sufficient. What should be the goal of an income maintenance or security system—100 percent replacement of past earnings? 50 percent? 70 or 80 percent? or perhaps 110 percent in times of inflation? How should the social security goal be achieved? Should it be universal in scope, requiring full participation of all workers and employers? Should it consist of a social insurance, earnings-related system exclusively, or should it be a two-tiered system involving both age requirements and past earnings and work history? Should it be mandated, as in France, that all employers provide a private pension scheme in addition to the social security system? Should a social security system provide for partial and more flexible pensions, permitting a mix between part-time earnings and partial pension income? This approach is being tried in Sweden for those between sixty and sixty-five years of age. Should it be based on a concept of shared equity and entitlement between husband and wife, with both spouses having accounts in their own right? Should today's social security schemes recognize homemaking and child-care responsibilities as having an economic value, much as in the open market? Job sharing and other emerging family life-styles need to be addressed if future elderly women are not to be condemned to a lesser and impoverished life. The policy issues related to the very old and women in old age are two of the most critical. They must be addressed by sound and innovative policies, and from a life span rather than an isolated life-stage basis. Such major policy questions are receiving particular scrutiny in the more developed countries as they attempt to relate social security to a changing world.

Stanford G. Ross (1979) identifies several major issues confronting social security worldwide. Included are financing problems based on "unfavorable demographic developments involving a declining number of contributors relative to an increasing number of pensioners," a problem confronting all the major industrialized countries. Ross notes:

> The aging of European populations has been proceeding at a much faster pace than in the United States. . . . The ratio of contributors to pensioners, which is 3:1 presently in the United States, is often lower abroad. Some advanced countries already have only about two contributors for every beneficiary; and there, like here, the projections are that the ratios will become even less favorable to pay-as-you-go systems as we enter the second and third decades of the 21st century (p. 6).

To deal with this, policymakers are attempting to develop mechanisms to encourage people to work longer, either by increasing the monetary incentives through pension increments or through gradually extending the retirement age. However, this strategy works at cross-purposes to the escalating demands of many trade unions for a lower retirement age, in order to make badly needed jobs available for large numbers of unemployed youth. Perhaps they are right: a full employment policy strategy for all ages might not only provide more payments into the social security system, but also better protect future generations of the aged from economic need.

In fact, in a developed society like our own, the idea of retirement seems increasingly anachronistic. Ross, for example, points out a radical difference in viewpoints on retirement between developed and developing societies:

> The idea of "retirement" as an abrupt termination of one's working life is increasingly viewed as appropriate only in relatively poor societies, where people work extremely hard in physically demanding occupations. Industrialized societies have developed to the point where people who choose to do so should be able to adjust their occupations to remain active in the elderly years (p. 7).

Such discrepencies in viewpoint lead to major policy questions at the international level. One such issue in the development of social policies is whether to use the situations and values of industrialized countries as the models for social policy programs elsewhere. For example, in many societies, income security for the aging may be of a lesser priority than providing a standard of subsistence income for all in the developing world. Similarly, a major concern may not be the changing of dietary requirements of older persons, but rather access to food for the entire population on a daily basis. As Simon Bergman (1981), borrowing from the Maslowian concept of a hierarchy of human needs, has pointed out:

> The developing countries, in regard to aging, are now at the level of having to meet the *most basic* needs of *food*, shelter, and security for the elderly; this means satisfying the needs "to have" before the basis for *"to be"* can be reached. This is at a time when Western aged are in the stage of "being and of becoming," i.e., in the stage of development and self-actualization versus the stage of survival and maintenance in the developing countries.

Professor Lawrence Adeokun (1980) of the University of Ife, Nigeria, supports this view and points out: "It is to the extent that colonialism and modernization placed emphasis on the individual and correspondingly weakened the family that the welfare of the aged has suffered."

Recently, however, the dominance of developed nations as safe models for social policy has begun to recede in favor of a true global perspective. In 1982, the United Nations will hold a World Assembly on the Aging, a decision which has received overwhelming support among the less-developed countries, as compared to reluctant support on the part of the more developed countries, including the United States. This effort has stimulated other UN-related agencies to consider their roles and responsibilities in the development of international programs and national policies relevant to the aging in their sphere of interest. The World Health Organization has targeted for the year 2000 primary health care for everyone in the world, including the elderly, and has established a global program on health and the aging, with particular emphasis on the developing countries.

Such broad global programs are especially encouraging, since social policy for the elderly is too often viewed as separate from other public policies. Yet programs that focus upon fiscal, tax, energy, urban, rural, and family policies may have a greater impact on older persons than a single piece of social legislation focused solely on the aging. In addition, the United States must be more responsive to third- and fourth-world development needs and issues—in the name of self-interest as well as in the name of broader humanitarian concern. It is within the context of broad international policies that social policies and aging must be addressed. Indeed, aging must be viewed as an integral part of economic and social developments. Policies of all kinds take into account the continuing contributions of older persons to such development, as well as addressing the specialized needs of this growing segment of the world society. And it is up to the United States to assume a major role in supporting such international efforts.

REFERENCES

Adeokun, Lawrence A. 1980. "The Aged and Their Welfare in Developing Countries: Observations from Nigeria." In *Adaptability and Aging*, vol. 2. Paris: International Center of Social Gerontology.

Beattie, Walter M., Jr. 1978. "Aging: A Framework of Characteristics and Considerations for Cooperative Efforts between the Developing and Developed World." Unpublished paper, Expert Group Meeting on Aging.

Bergman, Simon, 1981. "Aging and the Developing Countries." In *Adaptability and Aging*, vol. 2. Paris: International Center of Social Gerontology.

Council on Environmental Quality and the Department of State. 1980. *The Global 2000 Report to the President: Entering the Twenty-First Century*, vol. I. Washington, D.C.: Government Printing Office.

Kii, Toshi. 1978. "Recent Extension of Retirement Age in Japan." *Aging International* 5:19.

Ross, Stanford G. 1979. "Social Security: A Worldwide Issue." *Social Security Bulletin* 42:3–10.

Sauvy, Alfred. 1979. "Unemployment, Populations and Pensions." *Newsletter of the International Center of Social Gerontology* 31:1.

The President's Commission on Pension Policy. 1980. *An Interim Report*. Washington, D.C.: Government Printing Office.

United Nations Fund for Population Activities. 1980. *1979 Report*. New York: U.N. Fund for Population Activities.

United States Department of Health and Human Services. 1980. *Social Security Throughout the World: 1979*. Washington, D.C.: Government Printing Office.

RELATED READINGS

Aging in the Eighties

Binstock, R. 1980. "A Policy Agenda on Aging for the 1980s." In *National Journal Issues Book*. Washington, D.C.

Brody, E.M. 1980. "Women's Changing Roles and Care of the Aging Family." In *National Journal Issues Book*. Washington, D.C.

Cain, L.D. 1976. "Aging and the Law." In *The Handbook of Aging and the Social Sciences,* edited by R. Binstock and E. Shanas. New York: Van Nostrand Reinhold.

Davidson, S., and T. Marmor. 1980. *The Cost of Living Longer: National Health Insurance and the Elderly.* Cambridge, Mass.: Ballinger Publishing Company.

Demos, J. 1978. "Old Age in Early New England." In *Turning Points,* edited by J. Demos and S. Bocock. Chicago: University of Chicago Press.

Feder, J.; J. Holahan, and T. Marmor, eds. 1980. *National Health Insurance: Conflicting Goals and Policy Choices,* Washington, D.C.: The Urban Institute.

Hayflick, L. 1976. "Biology of Aging." *New England Journal of Medicine* 295:1302–08.

Hayflick, L. 1980. "The Cell Biology of Human Aging." *Scientific American* 242:58–66.

James, E., and J. James, eds. 1971. *Notable American Women.* Cambridge, Mass.: Harvard University Press.

Marmor, T.; B. Gold; and E. Kutza. 1976. "United States Social Policy on Old Age: Present Patterns and Predictions." In *Social Policy, Social Ethics, and the Aging Society,* edited by B. Neugarten and R. Havighurst. Washington, D.C.: Government Printing Office.

Neugarten, B., and R. Havighurst, eds. 1976. *Social Policy, Social Ethics and the Aging Society.* Washington, D.C.: Government Printing Office.

Schorr, A. 1980. *Thy Father and Thy Mother: A Second Look at Family Responsibility and Family Policy.* Washington, D.C.: Government Printing Office.

Schuck, P.H. 1979. "The Graying of Civil Rights Law: The Age Discrimination Act of 1975." *The Yale Law Review* 89:27–93.

Scott, Anne F. 1970. *Women in American Life.* Boston: Houghton Mifflin.

Scott, Anne F. 1978. "What Then Is This American, This New Woman." *Journal of American History* 65:679–703.

Siegel, J.S. 1981. "Demographic Background for International Gerontological Studies." *Journal of Gerontology* 36:93–102.

Creativity and Aging

Aldridge, Gordon. 1955. "Training for Work with Older People." In *Education for Later Maturity,* edited by Wilma T. Donahue. New York: Whiteside & William Morrow Co.

Brunvand, Jan H. 1968. *The Study of American Folklore,* 2nd ed. New York: W.W. Norton & Co.

Dancy, Joseph Jr. 1977. *The Black Elderly: A Guide for Practitioners.* Ann Arbor: Institute of Gerontology, The University of Michigan/ Wayne State.

Gardner, John W. 1963. *Self-Renewal: The Individual and the Innovative.* New York: Harper & Row Publishers.

Hemphill, Herbert W., Jr. 1974. *Twentieth-Century American Folk Art and Artists.* New York: E.P. Dutton & Co.

Jones, LeRoi. 1971. *Blues People.* New York: Morrow.

Lindsay, Inadel Burns. 1975. "Coping Capacities of the Black Aged." In *No Longer Young: The Older Woman in America,* pp. 89–94. Ann Arbor: Institute of Gerontology, The University of Michigan/ Wayne State.

Lipman, J., and A. Winchester. 1974. *The Flowering of American Folk Art.* New York: The Viking Press.

Lovell, John, Jr. 1972. *The Black Song: The Forge and the Flame.* New York: MacMillan & Co.

Lyell, Ruth Ganetz, ed. 1980. *Middle Age, Old Age: Short Stories, Poems, Plays and Essays on Aging.* New York: Harcourt, Brace, Jovanovich.

McLeish, John A.B. 1976. *The Ulyssean Adult: Creativity in the Middle and Later Years.* New York: McGraw-Hill Ryerson.

National Council on Aging. 1977. *Arts and the Aging: An Agenda for Action.* Washington, D.C.: Government Printing Office.

Southern, Eileen. 1971. *The Music of Black Americans: A History.* New York: W.W. Norton.

Spicker, Stuart F., Kathleen M. Woodward, David D. Van Tassel, eds. 1978. *Aging and the Elderly: Humanistic Perspectives in Gerontology.* N.J.: Humanities Press.

Sunderland, Jacqueline T., ed. 1976. *Older Americans and the Arts: A Human Equation.* Washington, D.C.: National Council on Aging.

A Tribute to Longevity

Barrows, C.H., and G.C. Kokkonen. 1977. "Relationship Between Nutrition and Aging." *Advances in Nutritional Research* 1:253–98.

Behnke, John; C. Finch; and G. Moment, eds. 1978. *The Biology of Aging.* New York: Plenum Press.

Bergsma, Daniel, and David Harrison, eds. 1978. *Genetic Effects on Aging.* National Foundation March of Dimes Original Article Series, vol. XIV, no. 1. New York: Alan R. Liss, Inc.

Borek, C.; C.M. Fenoglio; and D. King, eds. 1980. *Aging, Cancer and Cell Membranes.* Advances in Pathobiology Series, vol. VII. New York: Thieme Stratton.

Burnet, Sir Mcfarlane. 1974. *Intrinsic Mutagenesis: A Genetic Approach to Ageing.* New York: John Wiley & Sons.

Comfort, Alex. 1979. *The Biology of Senescence.* New York: Elsevier.

Finch, C., and L. Hayflick, eds. 1977. *Handbook of the Biology of Aging.* New York: Van Nostrand Reinhold Co.

Kohn, Robert R. 1978. *Principles of Mammalian Aging.* Englewood Cliffs, N.J.: Prentice-Hall, Inc.

Lamb, Marion J. 1977. *Biology of Aging.* New York: John Wiley & Sons.

Liu, R.K., and R.L. Walford. 1972. "The Effect of Lowered Body Temperature on Lifespan and Immune and Non-Immune Processes." *Gerontologia* 18:363–88.

Masoro, E.J.; B.P. Yu; H.A. Bertrand; and F.T. Lynd. 1980. "Nutritional Probe of the Aging Process." *Federation Proceedings* 39:3178–82.

Ross, M.H. 1976. "Nutrition and Longevity in Experimental Animals." In *Nutrition and Aging,* edited by M. Winick, pp. 43–57. New York: Wiley.

Sacher, G.A. 1977. "Life Table Modification and Life Prolongation." In *Handbook of the Biology of Aging,* edited by C. Finch and L. Hayflick, pp. 583–638. New York: Van Nostrand Reinhold.

Schneider, Edward. 1978. *The Genetics of Aging.* New York: Plenum Press.

Young, V.R. 1979. "Diet as a Modulator of Aging and Longevity." *Federation Preceedings* 38:1994–1000.

World Perspectives on Aging

Ageing International. 1973. Washington: International Federation on Ageing.

Fry, Christine L. et al. 1980. *Aging in Culture and Society: Comparative Viewpoints and Strategies.* New York: Praeger.

Amoss, Pamela, and Steven Harrell. 1981. *Other Ways of Growing Old: Anthropological Perspectives.* Stanford: Stanford University Press.

Berdes, Celia. 1978. *Social Services for the Aged, Dying and Bereaved in International Perspective.* Washington, D.C.: International Federation on Ageing.

Binstock, Robert, and Ethel Shanas, eds. 1976. *Handbook of Aging and the Social Sciences.* New York: Van Nostrand Reinhold.

Bulletin on Aging. 1977. New York: Social Development Branch, Department of International Economic and Social Affairs, United Nations.

Cowgill, Donald O., and Lowell D. Holmes, eds. 1972. *Aging and Modernization.* New York: Appleton-Century-Crofts.

Cox, Frances M. 1977. *Aging in a Changing Village Society.* Washington, D.C.: International Federation on Ageing.

Dunham, Arthur et al. 1978. *Toward Planning for the Aging in Local Communities: An International Perspective.* Washington, D.C.: International Federation on Ageing.

Home Help Services for the Aging Around the World. 1975. Washington, D.C.: International Federation on Ageing.

International Association of Gerontology. 1962. *Aging Around the World.* New York Columbia University Press.

International Journal of Aging and Human Development. 1973. Farmington: Baywood Publishing Company.

Missine, Leo, and Bonnie Seem. 1979. *Comparative Gerontology: A Selected Annotated Bibliography.* Washington: International Federation on Ageing.

Myerhoff, Barbara G., and Andrei Simic, eds. 1978. *Life's Career-Aging: Cultural Variations on Growing Old.* Beverly Hills: Sage Publications.

Palmore, Erdman. 1980. *International Handbook on Aging.* Westport: Greenwood Press.

United Nations Department of International Economic and Social Affairs, 1978. *International Directory of Organizations Concerned with the Aging: Supplement.* New York: United Nations Department of Economic and Social Affairs.

INDEX

LIST OF CONTRIBUTORS

The Perspectives on Aging Lecture Series was held at Duke University, the University of Michigan, the University of Southern California, and the University of Washington, under the auspices of Colonial Penn Insurance Group, Philadelphia, Pennsylvania.

The following nationally known authorities participated in this topical series:

George J. Alexander, J.S.D.
Dean and Professor of Law
University of Santa Clara School of Law

James E. Birren, Ph.D.
Executive Director, Ethel Percy Andrus Gerontology Center
University of Southern California

Walter M. Beattie, Jr., Ph.D.
Director, All-University Gerontology Center
Syracuse University

313

Leonard Hayflick, Ph.D.
Professor and Director
Center for Gerontological Studies, University of Florida

Alan Jabbour, Ph.D.
Director, American Folklife Center
The Library of Congress

Harold R. Johnson
Director, Institute of Gerontology
University of Michigan

Alice J. Kethley, Ph.D.
Deputy Director, Institute on Aging
University of Washington

John A.B. McLeish, Ph.D.
Vice President
U-P Associates

George L. Maddox, Ph.D.
Director, Center for the Study of Aging and Human
Development
Duke University

Theodore R. Marmor, Ph.D.
Professor of Political Science and Public Health
Yale University

George M. Martin, M.D.
Professor of Pathology, Adjunct Professor of Genetics
University of Washington School of Medicine

Edward J. Masoro, Ph.D.
Professor and Chairman, Department of Physiology
The University of Texas Health Science Center at San
Antonio

John B. Orr, Ph.D.
Professor of Social Ethics and Director of School of Religion
University of Southern California

Erdman Palmore, Ph.D.
Chief of Medical Sociology, Department of Psychiatry
Professor of Sociology, Department of Sociology
Senior Fellow, Center for the Study of Aging and Human
Development
Duke University

Michel Philibert, Ph.D.
Director, Centre Pluridisciplinaire de Gerontologie
Université de Grenoble

May Sarton
Author

Anne Firor Scott, Ph.D.
William K. Boyd Professor of History
Duke University

James A. Standifer, Ph.D.
Professor of Music
The University of Michigan